The Hair Bible

The Hair Bible

The Ultimate Guide to
Healthy, Beautiful Hair Forever

Susan Craig Scott, M.D., F.A.C.S.
with Karen W. Bressler

NEW YORK · SINGAPORE

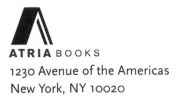

ATRIA BOOKS

1230 Avenue of the Americas
New York, NY 10020

This book is meant to educate and inform and should not be used as an alternative to appropriate medical care. For this reason, check the safety and efficacy of all medications and procedures with your doctor before using them.

A LifeTime Media Production
LifeTime Media, Inc.
352 Seventh Ave., 15th Floor
NY, NY 10001
President: Jacqueline Varoli
Editorial Director: Karen Kelly

Designed by Elissa Stein
Illustrations by Linda Anne Crank
Photos: Getty Images

ISBN 0-7434-4260-1

First Atria Books hardcover printing April 2003

10   9   8   7   6   5   4   3   2   1

ATRIA BOOKS and colophon are registered trademarks
of Simon & Schuster, Inc.

For information regarding special discounts for bulk purchases, please contact Simon & Schuster Special Sales at 1-800-456-6798 or business@simonandschuster.com

Printed in the U.S.A.

Contents

Introduction

Learning to live with or without your hair is a huge part of life. When we are born, we have very little hair, and soon it begins to grow into place. One of the first things we need to learn, in addition to how to walk, talk, eat, and speak is how to deal with our hair. Everyone's hair is different, so it's important for each of us to know the specifics of how our hair fits into our lifestyle.

We must become familiar with our hair type and learn how to care for it—when to shampoo it and when to "let it go" another day, how much conditioner to use and how long to leave it on, which brush to use and exactly when to start styling it.

My sisters inherited my mom's thick hair and they both have long, wavy manes. Always my father's daughter, I had to settle for pin-straight limp locks. The sibling rivalry started at an early age when we each wanted what the other had and it continues to thrive.

As we grow older, our hair grows too. Throughout our childhood, we choose the most decadent barrettes, ribbons, and bows and beg our moms to fasten them at the ends of pigtails and braids. Then we watch them spend hours on end trying to get the knots out after a long day at play. I will never forget that faithful bottle of No More Tangles sitting at the edge of the bathtub, ready and waiting to diligently go to work. For special occasions, my mom would set my stick-straight brunette locks in rollers and leave them in place overnight, only to unroll them the next morning and see the curls droop minutes later. Years of tap dancing lessons provided plenty of opportunities for carefully coifed 'dos that would take hours to undo at the end of each performance. We'd always find tiny flecks of silver glitter from our costumes strewn throughout our follicles.

Through it all, I was grateful that my generation did not have to endure what our mothers' and grandmothers' did. My mom, who grew up in the pre-blow-dryer era of the 1950s, remembers sitting under a hair cap with a hose attached to dry her hair. She wrapped her hair with toilet paper to straighten it and slept on hard curlers since softer versions were not yet available. In the 1960s her friends used falls, a sort of wig that let them wear their hair Hollywood style. My dad didn't approve of Mom sporting someone else's hair, so she grew her hair long, then cut it off and created her own fall.

My great-aunt tells stories of doing both her mom's hair and her daughter's. Her mom, my great-grandmother, had long silver locks, and my aunt used to set them in pin curls every night. Years later, before the flat iron was born, she slaved over an iron and ironing board trying to straighten her daughter's wildly curly mane.

So my life in relation to my hair seemed comparatively easier—I just had to get through it.

As the oldest of three daughters, whom my mom loved to dress alike, I was known as one of the Bressler sisters. Time and again our parents' friends and distant relatives failed to grasp the concept that we each had our very own individual first names. Things got worse when our mom started taking us to the same hair shop to get our haircuts. A famous photo that used to sit on our baby grand piano features all three of us and my mom with similar 'dos.

Class pictures were no fun either. I will never forget the night before my fourth-grade photo session when my mom took us to the local barber shop. My boyish pixie cut couldn't have happened at a worse time, and I'll always have the snapshot to remember it by.

Dorothy Hamill made the bob famous during my year in fifth grade, and of course I had to try it before deciding to let my hair grow to at least shoulder length. By the sixth grade, Barbra Streisand brought back the perm. The most popular girls in class, who probably had their own personal hairdressers, were the first to test-drive the new chemical concoctions and looked ultra-glam. But just my luck, I came out looking as if I'd stuck my finger in an electric socket. And there was no hiding it! By the end of first period, news of my afro was already circulating, and kids were stopping by my locker between periods to see the damage for themselves. In seventh grade, there wasn't one male classmate who didn't have the poster of Farrah Fawcett in her red bathing suit hanging above his bed, spotlighting—among other things—her golden blonde feathered-back mane.

Thank goodness for high school! (We would finally be allowed to express our individuality and wear our hair the way we wanted.) During my first semester, however, nothing prepared me for being chosen as a volunteer in the annual assembly for energy conservation. Little did I know that public humiliation was only seconds away as I was pulled from the audience, walked onto the stage in front of half the school, and gently placed my hand on the static electricity machine, only to have all the hairs on my head stand on end! The laughter was deafening.

During the next few years, my hair would undergo a series of extreme measures. Four years on the swim team (hundreds of laps a week in a chlorinated pool) were starting to take its toll. My hair turned tints of yellow, then green. My sisters and I tried every shampoo and conditioner under the sun. I remember being amazed at the fact that Body on Tap contained a healthy dose of beer. We turned to Wella Balsam and Pert to cleanse away our dirt and grime. We related to the Breck Girls as they bounced their beautiful locks across the TV screen. And we told two friends about the miracle of Faberge, and they told two friends, and so on and so on and so on. In the summers, we soaked in Sun-In and, when our mom put her foot down, we used real lemons instead. We "fed" our hair fattening egg yolks, vinegar, and mayonnaise because they were supposed to give us the beautiful, shiny, healthy hair that we dreamed of.

College was another era, and we couldn't wait to embrace it. Neither could our hair. Still eager to stand out in the collegiate crowd, I dragged my mom to the hair salon on a school break and made her watch as I let the colorist add what I thought would be subtle streaks. About twenty minutes into the process, my mom nervously screamed, "That's enough!" and I was whisked out of the salon. I didn't know the damage that had been done until a year later when the pledges in my sorority had to learn the names of all the founding sisters, of which I was one. One girl thanked me for making myself easy to remember. "You're the girl with the streak down the back of her head!" she said.

My first job after college was in the bookings department of *Vogue* magazine. I envied the models who had their hair done beautifully as a career perk and admired the stylists I booked for shoots who were able to make them look good. I was introduced to the top stylists in New York and began to learn about the skills and techniques that are available in this big city.

I became good friends with Michele Brothier of Filles et Garçons where I would go for cuts, color, and the very regular blow-dry. I entrusted my locks to Carmine and Beth Minardi who cut and colored my hair every six weeks to ensure that it remained on par with New York's tough fashion standards. And I attempted to "do" my 'do myself, in preparation for professional gigs like press parties and TV appearances as well as personal plans like weddings and dates.

I became the benefactor of an unending supply of beauty products as each day at work brought about a delivery of some sort. My friends began calling me all the time, eager to try out the latest and greatest concoction. I've had my hair snipped and analyzed and I've even had a microscopic picture of my cuticle blown up and presented to me in a silver Pottery Barn frame along with a complete breakdown of its health.

Always of the low-maintenance variety, I could get ready to go out in about 20 minutes, so I never understood friends who needed an hour to blow-dry their hair. I couldn't comprehend women who planned their days around their hair, missing sessions at the gym to make a blow-dry last or not hitting the beach to preserve their curls. As long as I have my Jennifer Aniston–inspired layers, I can get through the day.

As I grow older, it is even more difficult for me to understand the plight of my friends who have been slowly losing their hair naturally or those few who are undergoing chemotherapy and have had to watch their hair fall out. For someone who always thought of my roots showing as a major catastrophe, I realized I had a lot to learn about hair.

It is for this reason that I find a need for *The Hair Bible,* a comprehensive book on hair, how it grows, how we need to take care of it, and how we can deal with losing it. I believe all women will be able to relate.

Our hair is our best accessory, but it can also be our worst nightmare. I hope to quell that possibility by touching on the basics of hair care and offering advice from the most reputable professionals in the field and from individual women who share their inspiring experiences with us all. Enjoy!

Karen Bressler
New York, NY

Acknowledgments

Special thanks to Filles et Garçons, Allure Day Spa and Hair Design, and Minardi Salon in New York City for always being there to answer a last-minute hair question, offer a location for a photo shoot, or provide firsthand experience of the latest hair trends and techniques. Thanks also to Ken Paves, stylist, Profiles Agency in Los Angeles; Linda Banner, Ph.D., head of the Sexual Health and Medicine Program at UCSF and Stanford University; Oz Garcia, nutritional consultant and author of *The Healthy-High Tech Body*; Philip Kingsley Trichological Institute, New York, NY; Prive, Los Angeles, CA: Laurent D., stylist, Christopher, colorist, and Amanda George, colorist; Sally Kravich, bicoastal certified natural health expert; The Makeup Design Studio, New York: Kathy Pomerantz, makeup artist; Tova Salon, Beverly Hills, CA: Carrie White, creative director and hairstylist; Julian Ferrer Salon, New York, Julian Ferrer, owner. In addition, many thanks go out to the publicists who made access to all of the hairstylists, colorists, and medical experts that much easier: Anne Hardy Public Relations; Behrman Communications; Cairns & Associates; Canaan Public Relations; Chris Molinari; David Granoff Public Relations; Devries Public Relations; Diane Terman Public Relations; DNA Public Relations; Edelman Public Relations; Erika Somerfeld, founder, The Beauty Channel; Factory Communications; Kip Morrison, LaForce and Stevens; Lane and Coady; Lauren Kahn, Lippe Taylor Public Relations; Madeline Johnson, Magnet Communications; Marina Maher, Morehouse Communications; M. Booth & Associates, Inc.; Muse Public Relations; Nora Lawler; Phyllis Klein and Associates; Shop PR; Siren Public Relations; Susan Magrino Agency; Suzanne Bersh; The Brooks Group; The Professional Image; Tractenberg & Co.; Whisper PR.

Special thanks also to the people at LifeTime Media, Inc., including Jacqueline Varoli, Karen Kelly, and Lara Asher and to the people at Simon & Schuster, including Wendy Walker. Special thanks also to Tracy Bernstein.

Karen Bressler thanks "her mom, for making me 'Erma,' a self-named style that carried me through plenty of family occasions before I turned six; my grandmother Roslyn, who loved to braid my hair whenever I visited; my grandmother Rose, who always said, "Put your hair back so I can see your face"; Myrtle, who's an inspiration in gray; Marcia, who's always in style from hair to toe; my sisters Cindy and Suzanne—I always coveted their wavy hair and they wanted my straight 'do; and my Tante Jean, who is thankful I finished this book so I can give her hair advice in return for all the great advice she's given me over the years."

Dr. Susan Craig Scott thanks her husband, Dr. Norman Scott, and her children Eric, William, and Kelly. She would also like to thank New York Liberty and her many patients who over the years have taught her so much.

Part One
Your Hair

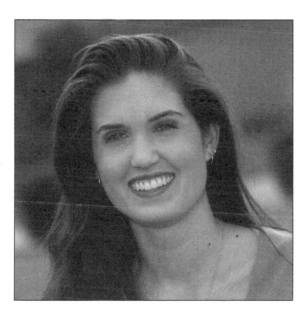

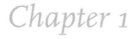

The Life of Hair

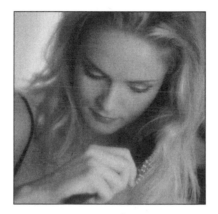

Hair. We brush it, blow-dry it, iron it, style it, shampoo it, condition it, color it, straighten it, curl it, perm it, pull it back, braid it, part it, section it, and subject it to salt water, chlorine, smoke, pollution, heat, humidity, and sweat. It is an integral part of our daily routine and we are constantly doing something to affect it.

To sustain our obsession with hair, there are thousands of hair salons around the world, making it a multibillion-dollar business. At some of New York City's top salons, like Elizabeth Arden and Frédéric Fekkai, women schedule appointments weeks in advance to see the stylist of their choice and pay hundreds of dollars to get the look they want. But regular cut and color visits are just the beginning of the maintenance process. More and more specialty clinics, where individualized hair care is the focus, are replacing traditional salons. A visit to the Philip Kingsley Trichological Clinic begins with an analysis and case history, nutrition advice, and a discussion of hair care, treatments, product lines, and follow-up counseling sessions via the phone. Physicians are consulted if a medical problem occurs. Why are we so concerned with our hair? Because it frames the face and it makes a strong first impression. It can embody beauty, power, attraction, age, grace, and health. Perhaps the most compelling characteristic of hair is that it is one of the few "accessories" that is attached to us on such a visible plane. Since our hair is such an obvious component of our appearance, it instantly becomes a statement of how well we take care of and how we view ourselves. People assume that our hair looks the way we want it to look or that we don't care how it looks. So others can pretty accurately assess the state of our confidence, organization, and well-being from the state of our hair.

Different hairstyles and colors represent a range of personality traits. A recent Yale University study, commissioned by Physique Hair Care, rated 300 images of men and women. The results were telling: Hair pulled back conveys intelligence, long dark curly hair is seen as outgoing, people with medium-length casual styles are deemed good-natured, and short hair signals confidence. Sexiness is associated with long, straight blond hair. The stigmas and character traits people match with hair have blossomed over time and remain with us wherever we go. Even further, women have proven that hair is one of the single most important aspects of their appearance due to its malleability. It can be changed quickly to help us accomplish a number of feats: starting over in a job or relationship, making it look as if we're on top of things, and temporarily covering other physical or emotional issues we don't want people to notice. For thousands of years, hair has been a powerful tool for our instant self-confidence, as well as a strong contributor to our lack thereof.

A History of Hair

Some of the first references to hair care appear as early as 4000 B.C., when Egyptians crafted combs out of dried fish bones. In 2000 B.C., Egyptians mixed water and citrus juice to make shampoo, and they applied animal fats and plant oils to their hair for conditioning. In 1800 B.C., Babylonian men powdered their hair with gold dust, and in 1500 B.C., Assyrian slaves curled the hair of kings and other nobles with heated iron bars. In 500 B.C., hair styling was born in western Africa, where sticks and clay were used as early versions of curlers and setting gel. Accessories and color were introduced in 35 B.C., when Cleopatra wore jewel-studded ivory pins in her hair and Roman prostitutes were forced to dye their hair blond. In the first century A.D., hair color became even more prominent. Women attended Roman feasts showing off their dark, shiny tresses,

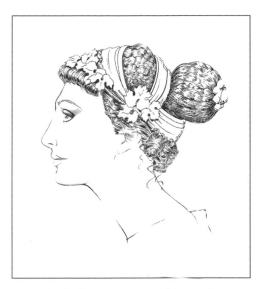

Ancient women managed to create elaborate hairstyles without the help of today's modern products.

thanks to dyes, which were created from boiled walnuts and leeks. Saxon men charged on the battlefield toward their enemies with their hair blazing in threatening hues of blue, green, and orange, in the year 100. In Rome, circa 200, sculptors began to attach marble wigs to their artwork to update them in accordance with the hairstyles of the times. And in the fourth century, there was an emphatic show of hairnets and scarves.

Fast-forward a millennium: If you think that permanent solution now smells awful, empathize with European women in the 1300s who conditioned their hair with dead lizards boiled in olive oil. And that's not all they had to endure; they also shaved their hairlines to show off high foreheads and piled hair high on their heads to make their necks look longer. We find it difficult today to meet society's physical ideals as projected by television, magazines, and other forms of media. Imagine the challenge women had in the 1400s, when the somewhat devious theoretician Machiavelli announced the standard for appealing locks, claiming that a woman should be crowned by hair that is "loose and blond, sometimes the color of gold, at other times honey, shiny as the rays of the sun, wavy, thick and long, scattered in long curls, and fluttering on the shoulders." Women who strictly adhere to the doctrines of some religions may relate to the married women of 16th-century Italy, who were expected to cover or braid their hair in the interest of modesty. Around the same time, French women frizzed their hair with heat and then sculpted it to towering heights. Red hair and wigs were made fashionable in England by Queen Elizabeth, and "blonding" was a hit, with a homespun dye composed of wine, spices, and herbs.

Finally, an entrepreneur capitalized on hair's phenomenal importance, paving the way for the Vidal Sassoons and Bumble and Bumbles of our times. In 1635, the very first ladies' hair salon, appropriately named Champagne, opened in Paris, France. Extra-firm-hold hair gel would have been an essential commodity in the 18th century, when stiff pompadours—masses of hair combed high, frizzed above the forehead, and held in place with paste and glue—were the rage. The entire period marked the origins of hairdressing as a true art form. Hairdressers constructed monuments out of hair as fashion statements, and even further, as statements about current events and deep emotions. The masterpieces were so elaborate that ladies reportedly had to crouch on their knees to fit the huge 'dos into their carriages as they traveled. Hundreds of years before the punk rock era as we know it, hair was powdered in blue, violet, white, pink, and yellow pastels.

Eventually, the rigidity gave way to a historic form of "bedhead."

These elegantly neglected styles featured disarrayed locks whimsically arranged and loosely tied, with overflows of curls in chocolate brown hues. Hair was also crimped, tousled, and caught up in chignons, with locks framing the face, much like today's special-occasion updo. Women also wore their hair knotted low in heavy chignons and accented with flowers. Late in the century, the French Revolution called for shorter, less elaborate styles. During the early 19th century, hats, hoods, and headdresses became popular in France. Plain and plaited hair made waves in England in the 1850s. The "'60s" were a different kind of groovy, with clip-on hair and big hair marking another change from the norm. In the 1870s, beauty parlors opened in the United States, featuring centennial chignons and dainty bunches of curls. In the 1880s, women charted the course for Crystal Gayle, wearing their hair all the way down their backs, even to the ankles.

The first signs of consumer distress with less tress came in 1900, right alongside a public striving to achieve the "ideal" figure. While corsets were drawn tighter than ever, chignon fillers like braids and swatches were wrapped around thin hair coils to resemble fuller heads of hair. Creative invention didn't stop there; it only flourished. As in many other fields, the 20th century brought invention to the hair industry that dramatically changed everything. In 1907, the first chemical hair color formula was born—named Aureole by its originator, Eugene Schueller, and then later rechristened L'Oréal. Charles Nestle invented the first permanent-wave machine in 1905. Madame C.J. Walker began selling hair care products for African-Americans in 1906, which later became a multimillion-dollar business. In 1917, the double-process blonding technique was invented, giving blondes worldwide more fun than ever!

Inspired by the vacuum-cleaner hose, the first hair dryer was invented in 1920, blowing away the old air-drying methods. By 1925, there were already 25,000 beauty parlors in the United States! Breck International set up shop in the 1930s. Sisters Maria and Rosie Carita opened a beauty salon in Paris in the 1940s. Present-day conditioner was created in the 1950s, when chemists discovered that ingredients used in fabric softeners could also soften hair.

The aerosol spray can was invented in 1956, making hair spray possible—and, therefore, probable. Redken popularized pH-balanced and protein-enriched shampoos for better conditioning in the 1960s. In 1971, the first hand-held blow-dryer limited trips to the salon by making it easy to simply "blow and go," and a special iron was invented in 1972 by Geri Cusenza that crimped—but did not cramp—anyone's style.

Hairstyles underwent rapid changes in the 20th century as well. Styles of the times reflected what was happening socially and were most often worn by icons of popular culture, which epitomized our ideals and our dreams.

Until, and through, the early 1900s, wealthy women had set the standard, donning hair jewels, bone combs, and veiled hats with lace, flowers, and feathers by day, and dusting their hair with silver and gold powders by night. A new look, created by Antoine of Paris, showcased hair parted in the middle and swept back in smooth bands over the ears. Edith Wharton sported a loose, wavy, poufy feminine look that also turned heads. In 1907, Josephine Baker's sleek style and the Marcel wave cascaded over the United States and Europe. By 1910, American nurses in Europe had fed a copycat trend back home. They had cut their hair short to protect themselves from flea infestation and women in America began to do the same for fashion.

Louise Brooks's 1917 bob became the most popular hair trend of the 1920s as women strove to express their freedom, shedding their corsets and entering the work force. The 1930s and 1940s found wartime citizens ogling the glamorous life. In 1931, Jean Harlow starred in *Platinum Blonde* and a hair color craze soon swept the nation and beyond. Also in the 1930s, child star Shirley Temple's tight curls had grown women pinning their hair into ringlets. During the war, when the feminine ideal was largely expressed through movies and film magazines, women copied Hollywood hairdos. In the 1940s, Rita Hayworth made side-parted finger waves the sexiest style of her time, and Veronica Lake's cascading blond hair redefined glamour.

By the 1950s, highlighting was the driving trend and so was Lucille Ball's flaming mane. Doris Day's helmet-hair inspired her fans, and Audrey Hepburn's role in *Roman Holiday* mobilized the modern pixie cut. Brigitte Bardot's "sauerkraut" (a.k.a. *choucroute*), a structured yet wavy 'do, was the one to emulate. Clairol's "Does She or Doesn't She?" advertising campaign reassured women that it was acceptable to color their hair. Housewives had a staid role in our 1950s and '60s society, and their hairstyles revealed that fact. In the '50s, the homemaker's hairdo was conservative, and in the '60s, women wore stiff Dynel wigs and toyed with the idea of wearing falls for Supremes-inspired styles. Toward the end of the era, beehives and bouffants became popular with the availability of hair spray and the trend toward a more carefree lifestyle.

The freedom of the 1960s was expressed even in popular hairstyles. People let their hair down and there was a distinct movement toward trading gender norms in hairstyles. British rock sensations the Beatles wore their hair long, a style generally out of fashion since the 19th century. Female model Twiggy wore hers short and boyish in a no-fuss fashion that abruptly ended the harsher '50s styles.

In 1963, Vidal Sassoon started issuing easy, wash-and-dry looks. Nearing the end of the decade, hair was also worn naturally long with little or no preparation, symbolizing liberation on many fronts for men and women.

In the 1970s, the musical *Hair* hearkened back to the rebellious lifestyle and sexual revolution of the late 1960s and early '70s, and Angela Davis's Afro became a symbol of black pride. Extremes like Grace Jones's forceful box cut and frosted wings defined the disco look, while Gloria Steinem's simple straight hair with a center part offered an anti-style statement. In 1974, the feathered hair of *Charlie's Angels* star Farrah Fawcett was the decade's most copied 'do. Variations of African-American braids were popularized in 1975, and Dorothy Hamill's short, layered wedge became a sporty trademark in 1976 after she won the Olympic gold medal for figure skating. But even as Dorothy spun, punk rock brought purple, blue, green, and orange Mohawks into focus. Cornrows were a "10" in 1979, à la Bo Derek.

In the 1980s, those newly prosperous from the economic boom opted for mall bangs, poodle perms, and voluminous hair. But Melanie Griffith showed that the first step on the woman's career ladder involved the shortening and taming of such "big" hair in the hit '80s movie *Working Girl*. Lady Diana's 1981 wedding made commoners around the world realize that dreams do come true if you have a short, elegantly layered head of hair. In 1988, Sinead O'Connor's shaved head, combined with her soft features, paved the way for all quiet, modern renegades, and dreads went glam as singer Lauryn Hill hit the charts that same year. Superstar Madonna started a revolutionary career with her controversial lyrics and stage moves and her wild, long, sometimes choppy, highlighted, root-infested tresses. The pop star exemplified a woman's right and capability to change her appearance as often as she liked, as was evident in the endless hair colors and styles she sported throughout the decade and beyond.

Change was the mantra of supermodel Linda Evangelista in the early 1990s. Because she constantly varied her hair's hue, length, and style, Linda's pictures in national women's magazines and her struts down designer catwalks were always anticipated. Anti-pop became popular itself in the 1990s, and grunge rocker Courtney Love's dark-rooted platinum look started the 1990s off with a screaming rant. By 1994, more conservative masses had found their "friend" in Jennifer Aniston's layered, angled shag cut. In the late '90s, middle-parted, quick-styled, long, straight, pale blond hair rose to stardom on the heads of Carolyn Bessette Kennedy and Gwyneth Paltrow, perhaps in response to the 1995 international agreement to eliminate the production of chlorofluorocarbons found in aerosols, such as hair spray cans. At the turn of yet another millennium, actress Sarah Jessica Parker graced the small screen in an award-winning show, prompting a widespread adoption of her flowing, curly locks.

What Your Hair Says About Your Personality

From work to play, hair reveals a lot about how we perceive ourselves and how others view us. The right haircut, color, and style can take us to the top of the career ladder or to the altar, or can help us accomplish any of our professional and personal goals.

"Hair has two roles in the workplace," says Paula Jaye, principal partner, Esposito/Jaye Associates, a New York–based management consulting firm. "First, it should project the image you want to achieve. If you work in a conservative environment, your hair should not draw attention to itself but blend in with the rest of your style. Go for a clean, crisp, well-put-together hairdo. If you work in the arts, media, or advertising, you can take more leeway and let your hair make more of a statement. Secondly, hair is directly connected to self-confidence. When hair is in good shape, beautifully cut, correctly colored, and you feel good about it, you will project confidence and grace. If your work is people-based and you are continuously meeting new clients, interacting with internal clients, and going to meetings, then having the right hairstyle can make you feel more confident." Adds Jaye, "Keep in mind, however, that great-looking hair is just icing on the cake. It's no substitute for having competence, skills, and the right technological background. But if all of these factors are in place, great hair will allow you to project more confidence as you deliver your message."

"No one ever has a bad makeup day, only a bad hair day," says Kathy Pomerantz, a New York City–based makeup designer. "And because hair is such a major factor in how we present ourselves, it's the first thing we change when we're ready for a new look." We change our hair when we start a new job, end a relationship, or attend a special event. We even change our hair when we want to showcase a different part of our personality. And sometimes the way our hair looks changes our personality without our realizing it. "The emotional relationship we have with our hair and the way in which it ties in with our personality is fascinating," says Ouidad, a New York City curly hair specialist. "Sometimes our hair is tamed, controlled, elegant, or easy, but sometimes it's wild and uncontrollable. If we are uncomfortable with its appearance, we can exude a sense of insecurity." Ouidad explains that unruly hair can cause subconscious mental discomfort, something that is obvious with curly hair that needs a lot of maintenance to control. She says even top lawyers feel they can't argue a case if their hair isn't done, and she cites a professor at Harvard who wears her hair pulled back while lecturing so students don't get distracted by her curls. Ouidad believes curly haired women have an advantage since they can change their hair from curly to straight with a simple blow-dry and therefore change their entire personality. Yet, interestingly enough, most women turn a cold shoulder to the concept of utilizing modern technology to permanently straighten their curly locks. "Once you take away a woman's right to constantly fight her hair, she feels like she has nothing to fight for anymore," explains the stylist. "Women won't part with their curly hair because they are afraid they will lose part of their personality and a sense of who they are in the process."

Hair color also plays a role in defining a woman's personality, according to a 1997 university research paper by experimental psychologist Dr. Tony Fallone, as cited in the *Vogue Book of Blondes*. The study indicates that blondes are more likely to be outgoing and lively and are perceived as more feminine than their brunette or redhead counterparts. Blond is not a color but a state of mind. The study continues that brunettes know allure because mystery is their secret weapon, but blond sexuality incorporates innocence and naïveté. Gentlemen, says Dr. Fallone, prefer blondes but marry brunettes.

"Hair is crucial to our state of mind," says Aleta St. James, emotional healer in New York City. "And color is a tremendous indicator of energy. If our hair is the wrong color, or a shade that doesn't complement our skin tone, we can feel uncomfortable about ourselves and not know why. When it's the right color and complements skin tone, we feel a sense of buoyancy and lightness that can lift our self-esteem. Any woman who's been through a situation where her hair colorist messed up on the formula, or her stylist has given her a bad haircut, understands this."

According to St. James, brunettes who change to red can feel livelier, and redheads who opt for deeper shades of brown can feel more subdued. "While sometimes red hair needs to be toned down and less flamboyant, turning a redhead into a brunette can make her feel like her light went out," explains St. James. The same applies to blondes. Darkening naturally blond hair can make a woman feel constricted, just as turning a brunette who wants to remain understated into a blonde can make her uncomfortable.

"Hair color should enhance a person's inner spirit and complement their color palate, which very decisively determines mood," says St. James. The same holds true for hair's cut and style. "When hair gets too heavy and starts dragging, it's easy to feel like we are dragging or feel droopy. And cutting hair really short can upset a lot of women. If a hair stylist isn't listening to what we're saying, it can really be upsetting. A bad haircut can also make us feel like staying home or wearing a hat until our hair grows out. Hair is an essential way in which we present ourselves, especially since it frames our face where most of self-expression takes place and where we communicate from."

None of us can imagine the impact that hair has on our self-perception and self-esteem until it doesn't live up to our expectations. A Yale University study conducted in the year 2000 showed that self-esteem and sociability of both men and women suffer when their hair is not at its best. According to the results, people feel less intelligent, less capable, more embarrassed, and less sociable. Men are more likely to be affected by a bad hair day than women are.

Jeffrey Paul, founder of Beautiful Hair Institute in Cleveland, Ohio, works with cancer patients and women who have lost hair due to other factors, says research shows that one out of every five women has hair problems that are not resolvable in the salon. In most cases, he believes women feel the loss of hair is greater than the disease itself. "Media projects what beautiful hair should look like, and women who don't achieve it will sense their emotional levels drop," says Paul. "This type of cosmetic stress affects women's hormones, which in turn affects hair loss. Her immune system drops, and she can become weak, depressed, and more vulnerable to acne and other sicknesses. When put into perspective, it's easy to recognize that it's only hair we're talking about. But it's really not. Hair defines a woman's frame, femininity, sexuality, and personality, and when pieced together properly in the overall image puzzle, it can make someone feel complete, whole, beautiful. People who are concerned with their hair constantly struggle with stress and spend tons of money trying to adjust. After all, one can't achieve inner beauty until she feels comfortable on the outside."

Hair Health

The quality and appearance of hair is influenced by overall health and diet as would be expected. Anorexics who starve themselves often have very fine, brittle hair, deficient in various minerals. Hair conveys information about a person and their state of health; further analysis of the hair can also tell what drugs they have taken. Long hair obviously suggests at least a recent history of good health.

"When I put people on diets one of first things they notice is the change in the quality of their hair," says Sally Kravich, a certified natural health expert who has traveled around the world studying longevity. "There is a certain sheen and quality of thickness to it. The typical American diet of foods with little or no nutritional value directly affects hair, skin, and nails. We don't get enough vegetables, whole grains, or good oils like avocado and olive oil, which can really make a difference. Instead, we load up on artificial sweeteners and diet sodas, which are some of the first products to make our hair fall out. And people think good hair is sexy, so if it looks bad, it's really noticeable."

MYTH: Keeping hair clean on a daily basis is all that's required for healthy hair.

FACT: Washing hair daily isn't enough for most adults. Proper conditioning, brushing and combing, styling, and other treatments do help hair maintain its health and appearance. Knowing the right treatments and techniques makes the difference.

"Once hair is damaged," says Kravich, "there is no quick-fix pill, only combinations of the right vitamins and a proper diet that will restore hair's natural health, volume, and luster." Just like an animal's coat, which looks healthier if the animal eats foods that are high in nutrients, minerals, and oils, basic things that will help hair include B-complex vitamins, minerals, and calcium to add thickness and shine. "Hair problems can also result from an unbalanced thyroid or hormonal changes, as in pregnant women," says Kravich. "Pregnant women are advised to take prenatal vitamins, but they don't always offer enough of what we need, such as folic acid."

The fitness craze that has been booming since the '80s has brought about a demand for a woman's hairstyle to complement her lifestyle. Whether a woman is an avid exerciser or continually on-the-go, her haircut needs to be low maintenance and still look great. "Women are always in search of carefree hair," says stylist and salon owner Paul Labrecque, who operates his salon under the roof of New York's Reebok Fitness Club. "They want something that looks fabulous when you wash it, regardless of whether or not you roller-set it or blow-dry it."

To give women what they want, Labrecque cuts wavy hair to accentuate the wave and to make it the feature of the hair instead of trying to pull the wave out and straighten hair. He cuts straight hair into a swingy line so that the straightness shows. Fitness fanatics, he says, can either go short or wear stretch bands to hold hair back. Adds Labrecque, "If you have a haircut that needs a lot of maintenance, it can slow down your lifestyle. You won't be able to work out then go to dinner afterward because you will have to get ready for the second time that day. Women who live in cities move quite rapidly and don't have time for this. They go from work into workout mode to play mode all within two hours. They have to make sure they're not spending a lot of time changing their look." He adds, "When hair looks healthy, you feel more beautiful. When you look your best, others perceive you that way."

This is exactly why women make such a big deal over their hair on their wedding day. With a booming bridal business under her belt, Laura Geller, owner of Laura Geller Makeup Studio, New York City, knows the importance of wedding hair only too well. "Every bride sees her wedding day as a once-in-a-lifetime event, something she has thought and dreamed about all of her life," says Geller. "The last thing she wants is a bad hair day on her wedding day when she's in the spotlight. Hair is the first thing people see and it is the focus of the eye, especially if the bride wears a headpiece or veil." Geller explains that the combination of the texture, color, length, and style all create the finished look, so it is understandable that many brides go through a number of trials until they get it right. "When hair is sloppy, it doesn't sit well with the headpiece, or if the cut is bad, it shows in every picture," says Geller. "People always compliment the bride when her hair is done right, far more often than commenting on a beautiful makeup job."

The truth of the matter is, however, the groom will most likely still say "I do" whether or not every hair on his bride's head is perfectly in place. It's the guys who aren't roped in yet that could have a problem with the cut or color of a woman's coif. "If a woman has a gorgeous, striking head of hair, a guy will notice it right away," says Susan Rabin, M.A., who has a master's in counseling, and is the author of *101 Ways to Flirt* and the director of School of Flirting and www.schoolofflirting.com. "Men like long hair better than short hair because it has a more teasing, sexual look. Hair is a flirting device, especially if you flip it, twirl it, toss it, stroke it, put your hand through it, and give off a more sensual vibe."

Rabin, who cites Julia Roberts for her volume and Kim Delaney for her sometimes-curly, sometimes-straight locks as having head-turning tresses, explains that tousled hair can be sexier than hair that's set in its place. "Guys see this as a turnoff," she says, "a sign that a girl is high-maintenance and that she is too concerned with her appearance and not enough about what's going on in the relationship." Of course, adds Rabin, a certain amount of sexiness is obtained by good grooming—no one wants hair that's dirty or too messy. "Women change their hair color all the time to attract different guys," adds Rabin. "And if you get a bad haircut and don't feel good about yourself, you won't flirt as well."

Your sex life can also be at stake. "Men say hair can be really arousing," says Linda Banner, Ph.D., head of the Sexual Health and Medicine Program at UCSF and Stanford University, which focuses on identifying the effect of sexual arousal on the brain. "If a woman has long hair and it droops down creating a privacy veil that envelops the couple, intimacy can be more profound. Hair color can make a difference, too. Some men are turned on by redheads, some blondes, and others brunettes." What doesn't work: "Women who promote the don't-touch-me attitude, or are so absolutely proper they always have every hair in place. Sex is all about touch, so the fresh-out-of-bed look is important. Men and women want to run their fingers through their partner's hair. But if you're untouchable, your whole sexual experience can be inhibited. Sex is supposed to be spontaneous, pleasurable, fun, playful."

Some cultures consider women's long hair to be so sexually provocative that it has to be covered up. Tightly controlled hair, which has been rolled, curled, and sprayed, suggests a controlled woman, specifically one who controls her sexuality. "The more confident you are in general, the more self-esteem you will have," says Banner, "thereby enhancing your level of sexual pleasure and arousal."

Hair will continue to shape culture, as we strive to emulate the latest pop icons and celebrity style. But what if our hair just isn't conducive to the cut of the moment? What if it's too thin, thick, curly, or straight to make it do whatever is "in" at the moment? There are many tools of the trade that will help your hair to behave. After all, maintaining healthy hair is the most important aspect to achieving beautiful hair that works for you.

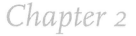

Chapter 2

How to Care for Your Hair

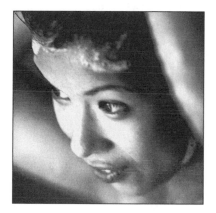

Our hair is the ultimate beauty accessory and one of our most impressive physical traits. And the most extraordinary thing about it is that no matter what we do to it, it keeps growing back (for most of our lives, anyhow, but we'll get to hair loss later).

What Is Hair?

The hair root originates deep in the dermis and grows up through the scalp, where it is called a shaft. The health of our hair depends on a healthy scalp. Too much oil (sebum) and sweat on the scalp can clog the follicle and inhibit healthy hair growth. Too little oil can cause the scalp to be dry and flaky. Each hair cuticle is made up of keratin and moisture. Keratin is the same protein that forms the base of nails, teeth, and skin. Vitamin deficiencies, illness, chemical processes, product abuse, and over-styling are some of the factors that can cause weak, lifeless hair. The cortex makes up 90 percent of the weight of the hair strand. It gives hair texture, strength, elasticity, and color, and it contains melanin, or pigment. The rest of the strand is made up of the cuticle, the outermost layer, and the medulla, the lightweight, air-filled core.

What's Your Type?

In order to know how to maintain healthy hair, it's important to determine your hair type. There are several factors to consider: First, is your hair

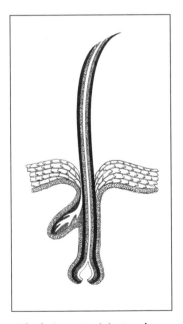

The hair root originates deep in the dermis and grows up through the scalp, where it is called a shaft.

straight, wavy, curly, or kinky? Remember, we're talking about the actual hair strand itself, not the texture your hair appears to have when the strands are styled together in one complete look. Straight hair usually has no curl and no wave. It's more likely to be oily than dry, either fine or thin, and super soft. Sometimes it can be medium textured with lots of body, or coarse and resistant to curling and shaping. Wavy hair is usually coarse, easy to handle, and can be blown out into straighter styles or worn curlier. It has a tendency to become frizzy. Contrary to popular belief, curly hair is often baby soft and fine and gets curlier or frizzier in humidity. It can be easily styled into a curly look or blown out into a smoother style. Curly hair has strong elasticity, so curls are usually shiny, soft, smooth, springy, and well defined. The longer and straighter curly hair is, the looser the curls. Shorter curly hair is often known for its tight, corkscrew curls. Kinky hair appears coarse but is really fine hair with thin strands packed together. It may feel silky but doesn't look shiny. The condition of your scalp also plays a role in determining your hair type. Overstimulation of the oil glands due to stress, vitamin deficiency, poor diet, and sweat gives your hair greasy clumps at the root, which can attract dirt quickly. The result: oily hair that usually can be remedied by shampooing often with a gentle shampoo. Dry hair is generally caused by a combination of genetics and environmental factors such as sun, salt, and chlorine, which make your scalp deficient in fatty acids or other nutrients. Overprocessing can also cause hair to look dull, break easily, get frizzy, or be prone to split ends. Use a moisturizing shampoo like one with wheat germ oil and a conditioner to bring your dry hair back to life. Maintaining a well-balanced diet and a gentle hair care routine will give you strong, soft, shiny hair that's full of body and easy to handle. Shampoo every other day or daily with a gentle shampoo to keep your hair looking great.

A Test for Your Hair

To help identify your hair type, pull a strand of hair from your head and perform these two tests. First, try to thread the hair through a needle as if you were threading it with string. If the hair slides right through, it's fine and probably straight. If you have trouble threading the needle or if the hair gets caught along the way, your hair is thicker and wavy or curly. Next, drop the hair into a glass of water. If the hair floats, it's either healthy or a bit oily since oil and water don't mix. If it sinks to the bottom, it's obvious that it absorbed a great deal of water to make up for the moisture it lacks, so it must be dry.

Got a Problem?

One of the most significant problems in caring for our hair is that, despite all the information we are provided with to help us determine our hair type, most women still don't know what their hair needs. Or they neglect giving their hair the treatment it requires out of laziness. "Most people don't condition or take care of their hair the way they should," says Ted Giza, senior stylist at the Avon Salon and Spa in New York City. "For example, straight hair needs to be washed and conditioned as much as curly hair, and flyaway static ends are a sure sign of hair that's void of moisture. Hair is an accessory. We wear our hair like jewelry or makeup. People should say, 'Wow, that's an elegant, beautiful woman' not 'Oh my god, her hair looks amazing.' If you are getting compliments on your whole look, you have successfully found the proportion, style, and texture that work well for you."

If you haven't quite figured out your personal hair care formula, consider some of these common problems that can be easily fixed to give you healthier hair. "One of the biggest mistakes women make is using the wrong products the wrong way," says Ted. "You'll know you're using the wrong shampoo and conditioner by the way your hair responds. If you use a detangler for dry hair, it will still be frizzy. If you use a heavy-duty conditioner on straight, fine hair, it will look greasy." In today's oversaturated market, it's easy to be confused about which products to use. "With hundreds of shampoos and conditioners out there, most will work for someone, somewhere, sometime. But just because one product works for your friend, doesn't mean it will work for you."

Another common hair problem is not cutting your hair often enough. "Split ends are the culprit," says Ted. "They tend to look frayed like fiberglass. A lot of women think they don't have to get haircuts while they are growing out their hair, but the longer hair becomes, the more ends split and you ultimately have to cut off more than you intended to. Regular trims help clean up splitting, especially if you blow-dry or style hair regularly."

Getting a proportionate haircut is also key. Ted says, "It's hard for women to learn to trust their stylists, because while they know they can probably give a technically good haircut, they may not always choose one that's right for their face. If you stop getting complimented on your hair, chances are it probably isn't the right cut or color for you."

Styling aids are another issue, and smoothing a dollop of gel onto your scalp isn't always the answer. "Most of us don't understand how styling products work," says Ted. "We don't know the difference between grooming and straightening balms, laminates or silicones, volumizers, mousses, or gels. We don't know what's meant for the hair shaft, hair ends, or roots. We apply a product to the wrong part of our hair and wonder why the ends are still frizzy, unkempt, and dull. More often than not, stylists don't educate their clients about products and too often even if they do, the clients are not really listening."

Washing, Brushing, and Styling

Proper hair care is part of your daily ritual and just as important as brushing your teeth or getting dressed in the morning. Your hair should be regularly washed, brushed, and styled in order to help it look and feel its best. Here is what you need to know to get through the basics.

Getting Serious About Shampoo

The sebaceous glands at the base of each hair shaft secrete oil. This oil, known as sebum, coats hair with a greasy layer that lubricates and softens but also attracts dirt and pollutants. Shampooing cleans both your hair and scalp by lifting dirt and oil. Sounds simple, right? Not so if you've stopped by a local drugstore lately and scanned the shelves in search of the right formula for you. Before you buy, decide what benefits you're looking for in a shampoo and it will be easier to narrow down the options and make your choice.

Obviously, the primary purpose of a shampoo is to cleanse our hair, but there are secondary benefits, like conditioning hair. "Two-in-one shampoos are conditioning shampoos designed to moisturize dry, damaged, or colored hair," explains Joanne Crudele, development manager for Unilever, the manufacturers of Salon Selectives, Finesse, Thermasilk, and Suave, among other brands. "For example, Salon Selectives is a hipper, trendier brand for more experimental women, Finesse is for women who want soft, beautiful hair, Thermasilk is a heat-activated shampoo that targets special styling needs, and Suave offers basic performance at a value-conscious price." Choosing a shampoo depends not only on the needs of your hair but also somewhat on your lifestyle. Women with dry, thick hair can tolerate shampooing every other day, since overshampooing can make their hair frizzy and bushy. Women with oily hair, or women who use lots of products in their hair, should shampoo at least once a day, sometimes even twice. It's important, however, not to overshampoo your hair. For example,

Is Your Hair in Condition?

To determine if your cuticle is damaged, shampoo and condition hair, then comb it out. If the comb sticks toward the end, the cuticle is damaged and you need a deep moisturizing conditioner. Some leave-in conditioners penetrate the cortex and build hair from the inside out.

curly hair tends to be on the dry side because it takes longer for oil to make its way down a curly hair shaft. If you shampoo curly hair more than two or three times a week, you run the risk of stripping hair of its natural oil, which seals and smooths the cuticles so that they reflect light and make hair look shiny. In addition, you will dry out the ends, which never get the benefit of the sebum. Most experts agree that shampoos with high levels of plant extracts buffer moisture loss and prevent hair from drying out.

Generally speaking, most women shampoo at least once a day using lukewarm water. The amount of shampoo you use varies according to the length and texture of your hair, but as a guideline, smooth a palmful into one hand and smooth it over your hair by starting at the scalp and stroking outward from root to tip instead of in a rough, circular motion, which can cause the hair fibers to rub together and tangle hair. Rinse in cool water to close cuticles and stimulate circulation to the scalp. Be sure to rinse well because product buildup dulls the hair. To dry hair, Crudele suggests using your hands as a squeegee to wring out the excess water, then lightly patting hair with a towel.

"Shampooing needs change as you age," says Crudele. "Hormonal changes in your body can slow hair growth, cause hair loss, or limit the production of natural lipids on the hair, which can make hair feel coarse. As you age, you may find you need to shampoo less so your hair doesn't feel overdry, or you may want to try a lighter-weight shampoo because you have less hair than you used to."

MYTH: For best shampooing results, choose a shampoo and stick to it.

FACT: Rotate shampoos to ensure that you get the best performance from each. The same shampoo doesn't work well after a while because your hair gets used to it. At the same time, you might require different benefits from your shampoo on different days. If you have less time to get ready one day, try a two-in-one shampoo. If your spirits need a lift another day, try an aromatherapy shampoo.

Get in Condition

Using a conditioner regularly helps improve the moisture content of hair and lock in that moisture so that it doesn't evaporate into the air. Conditioners leave a film of fatty acids and silicone on the hair to smooth the cuticle so that styling tools glide right through. As hair gets damaged, it soaks up conditioners even more. Conditioners help reduce the friction and static electricity caused by the interaction between hair strands. While most women condition their hair every other day, some fall victim to over- or underconditioning. Overconditioning can be caused by conditioning too frequently or by leave-in conditioners. "All conditioners leave some amount of product on your hair," says Cheri McMaster, a senior scientist at Pantene, "but a lightweight conditioner will leave less behind. Leave-ins can do wonders for thick hair that needs extra moisture but can weigh down fine, straight hair and leave it looking greasy." They are often available in liquid spray form, which can be directed onto a specific area of hair, such as the ends or a dryer patch where you need additional conditioner or shine. Leave-in conditioners are ideal for children who need help detangling messy locks, protecting hair from the elements, and restyling bedhead hair, which is popular among boys who don't want to take the time to do their 'dos. Two-in-one shampoos and conditioners save space in your bag when you travel and fit neatly into your locker at the gym, plus they can cost less than buying shampoo and conditioner separately. But if you really need a good conditioner, the two-in-one products probably won't do the trick. That's because the shampoo component adds surfactants for cleaning; surfactants increase the level of static electricity in hair, which defeats the purpose of using a conditioner.

Fun Hair Facts

- The average number of hairs is 140,000 for blondes, 100,000 for brunettes, and 90,000 for redheads.

- Hair grows about $1/2$ inch per month, faster in warmer weather.

- A healthy person loses 75–100 hairs per day.

- Each strand has a life cycle of two to seven years.

- Hair falls out to make room for new hair and the cycle starts again.

- The cuticle is made up of overlapping scales; healthy cuticles lie smooth and reflect light, which gives hair its shine.

To condition correctly, suggests McMaster, experiment with different amounts of product to find your own magical formula. A pea-size dose applied to the ends of fine, thin hair is appropriate. Thicker, coarser hair will eagerly soak up a capful of conditioner. "Focus on the ends and work your way up from tip to root," says McMaster. "For thick hair, work your hands right up to the scalp. Try not to let the product drip on your skin or it may cause your face to break out. Leave conditioner on your hair while you wash your body or shave so that it has time to make your hair smooth and shiny. The longer you leave conditioner on your hair, the better it works; five to ten minutes is ideal. For more protection, rinse with cool water so that some of the conditioner stays put even after you wash it."

To determine if your cuticle is damaged, shampoo and condition hair, then comb it out. If the comb sticks toward the end, the cuticle is damaged and you need a deep moisturizing conditioner. Some leave-in conditioners penetrate the cortex and build hair from the inside out.

Parting Ways

"You have to feel totally comfortable with where you part your hair," says New York City salon owner Julian Ferrer. "Otherwise, it never feels quite right." Style is also a consideration, according to Ferrer, who says there's a big difference in a haircut if your part is on the wrong side. "When the wind blows the hair, it won't fall in the right place; some pieces will look longer than others."

Ferrer confides that the trick is to cut hair with the part in the middle, then after finishing the cut, the hair should be recut on the side desired by the client. This is done so that when the style moves, the hair will always fall in lines that connect with each other. "A haircut should always have connection no matter where the part falls," says the stylist. "You want it to be even on each side, even if you part your hair differently one day." Changing your part from time to time can help maintain healthy hair. If you normally wear your hair parted to the right, and you move your part to the left, you can give fine, limp hair a little more lift without weighing hair down with gels, sprays, or other styling products. Says Ferrer, "Make use of the natural way hair falls. After a while, it becomes a habit and you can train hair to fall naturally into a certain position." Basically, says Ferrer, when parting hair, it's up to each individual to wear her part in a way that assures she looks good.

The Big Brush-Off

If you've been following Marcia Brady's advice all these years, you may be overbrushing your hair. The beauty-obsessed teen would make it a practice to brush her long, honey-colored locks 100 times a day. But the truth is, overvigorous brushing damages hair by stripping away the outer cells to expose the inner shaft, breaking brittle hair or dislodging hair that's not yet ready to depart. Overbrushing oily hair can supercharge the sebaceous glands and actually damage hair. Experts say a mere ten to twenty gentle strokes a day should do the trick.

The good news: Brushing encourages blood circulation, stimulates sebum-producing glands, distributes oils to give hair strands a silky coat, and dislodges dry scalp flakes, dust, and product residue. Brushing upward from the nape of the neck while bending forward adds volume after you flip hair back into place, but never brush hair when it's wet and at its weakest. Instead, "use a wide-tooth comb to comb hair out after shampoo," says celebrity hairstylist Steven Dillon, of the Gil Ferrer salon in New York City and beauty advisor for www.reflect.com. "Start at the bottom and work your way up to the roots to minimize any chance of getting tangles or breaking your hair."

Save Your Style

"Hair is the best accessory we have," says Ken Paves, of Profiles Agency in Los Angeles. "If our hair looks amazing, it doesn't matter if we're wearing sneakers and jeans or Manolos and a Prada suit. But if our hair doesn't look its best, it ruins the whole look." Paves says that when it comes to their hair, women should be able to charge things up a bit. "I love women who take risks and do things for the moment, such as adding extensions or clips or using a great product," says Paves, who swears by the hand lotion trick (a drop of hand lotion swiped across your hair will seal the ends and replenish moisture). Even distribution of lotion on towel-dried hair is also key. The most effective way, however, to keep your style intact is to use styling products correctly. "Most women put gel, mousse, or volumizer on their hands, then wipe their hands on top of their hair. The product usually doesn't make it to the underlayers or the ends. You need to apply a product in sections starting at the nape of your neck, and comb it through each section to distribute it from roots to ends (except root volumizer, which should be used only on roots) to get the maximum bene-fit. "Texture is the foundation of any look," Paves continues. "Setting your style with heat makes the cuticle expand and the shape of the hair shaft change, so it's important to let hair cool naturally before continuing to style. When the cuticle cools down and closes, the style locks into shape."

If you want straight hair, suggests Paves, be sure to go continuously through the motion of evening out the texture all over. If you use a blow dryer or straightening iron, allow hair to cool so that the texture will set and last longer. If you want a straight look with a slight bend at the ends, blow hair out with a dryer and a large-size round brush, then wrap hair around your head as if it was one big roller and let it cool to lock in the texture. If you're going for wavy hair, start with a good blow-out and wrap hair around a curling iron to make it wavy. Let hair cool, and then run your fingers through it to allow the style to set. "I love hair that moves, that's sexy, touch-able, and looks lived in—believable hair," says the stylist. "That's what's modern to me. It's all about what makes a woman feel the best about her-self, what makes her feel beautiful and sexy at this very moment in her life."

According to Paves, making a haircut look modern is as easy as bringing out a woman's eyes or hiding her high forehead—whatever makes her
feel sexy and confident. When going from the office to after-hours, Paves recommends starting with a sleek blow-dry and minimal products like a volumizer to add body or a defrizzer to smooth hair. Apply a moisture cream in the
evening for a more modern, sophisticated look. An off-center or side part is
less severe than a center part and will help create a more dramatic effect.

Down-to-Earth Issues

You can choose the right stylists and products, but you can't hide from
environmental factors that take a toll on your hair. Culprits can range from air
conditioning indoors to dry cabin air inside an airplane to sunlight or snow. But,
says Pat Peterson, director of research and development for Aveda, the most
harmful environmental factors are those you can actually see. "As long as there
are particles for your eye to see, as in steam or smoke, which are actually little
bits of ash surrounded by bits of gas that are floating in air, there is cause to take
cover. If your house was dusty, you'd cover the furniture," she explains. For
more information on how the environment affects our hair, see Chapter 6.

Scalp Salvation

"Since the scalp excretes sebum, which can leave hair fine and limp, it
needs to be cleansed, toned, and conditioned as hair requires," explains Rick
Goldberg, head coach for Progressive Beauty Brands, a company with hair care
products that contain tea tree oil, green tea, and lotus to treat the hair problems
in a natural, homeopathic way. If you have a dry, flaky scalp or dandruff,
advises Goldberg, use tea tree, which is antimicrobial, antifungal, and antibac-
terial by its inherent properties. Tea tree is also a natural inhibitor for children
who are exposed to lice. Green tea neutralizes free radicals and, according to
recent studies, acts as a UVA/UVB inhibitor so it can protect the hair and scalp
from the sun while maintaining vibrant hair color. The lotus flower, a Chinese
herb that can be found in some health food stores, has the appearance of luster

and sheen. It is the perfect remedy for dry or dull-looking hair since it helps balance the scalp, condition hair, and add sheen or shine.

Daily massage can help keep the scalp healthy by encouraging the flow of nutrients, thus preventing hair from falling out prematurely. For a quick daily massage, use fingertips to massage tiny circles from the nape of the neck to the forehead, and across the hairline. If your hair is oily, massage gently. If it is dry, massage more vigorously to stimulate oil glands. Brushing hair helps too, and, if you really want to have fun, a headstand every now and then keeps the blood circulating.

The Right Products: How to Pick, What to Mix

Shampoo

Ask yourself what specific benefits your hair type requires. Is your hair dry or damaged? Does it need more or less conditioning? Should you choose a clarifying shampoo to strip away residue that can build up on hair? Do you like the fragrance? Do you want a shampoo that will make your hair shine? Ingredients like macadamia nut, olive, jojoba oil, or shea butter have been used for years to give hair a shiny coat. Two-in-one shampoos are another option and ideal for women who want to save time, money, and space in their gym bags.

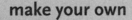

make your own

Shampoo: Skip the soap, which can dry both the hair and scalp and may contain chemicals that penetrate the bloodstream through hair follicles. Instead, add a few drops of lemon juice to your regular shampoo each time you wash or combine triple-strength herbal tea (chamomile for light hair, rosemary or sage for dark) ▶

▶ to an equal amount of your shampoo. You can also moisturize dry, brittle hair with vegetable oil to create an oil-enriched shampoo; add unflavored gelatin or an egg to your regular formula for a protein shampoo; or combine alcohol and water (1 to 3 parts) for a sudsless shampoo.

Conditioner

The most important ingredients to look for in choosing a conditioner are fatty acids. Look at the first five ingredients listed on the label and you'll see mentions of acetyl or stearyl alcohol and other ingredients ending in "amine," which are designed to combat static. A creamy-feeling formula, one that feels like a hand cream, will work best. It's also relevant to choose a conditioner that's designed for your hairstyle, like a volume conditioner to give hair a lift or a curl-enhancing conditioner to play up your curls.

make your own

Conditioner: Avocado adds protein and oil for shine and manageability. Egg yolk mixed with two teaspoons of castor oil and one teaspoon of rum moisturizes dry hair. Mayonnaise mixed with one beaten egg yolk and one teaspoon each of vinegar and powdered kelp adds shine and body. Honey, on its own, conditions any shade. Massage any of these natural conditioners into dry hair, cover with a shower cap, and allow to permeate for 30–60 minutes before shampooing. To speed up the process, wrap hot, moist towels around your head.

Gels, Sprays, or Mousses

Different products do the trick, according to your hair's texture. But here are some guidelines: Hair sprays work well for any hair type; choose one with a lighter chemical grade if you have fine hair that gets easily weighed down. Gels add texture, volume, and shine, increase holding power, control frizz, provide moisture, and smooth hair. Choose a lightweight formula for thin hair, save the extra-hold for thicker, wavier locks. The same rules basically apply for other styling products. Mousse is designed to increase hold and shine and combat static; choose a formula that can be easily brushed out so hair isn't sticky. Pomades increase the degree of hold, texture, and shine. Wax sticks add shine and help lock in moisture.

make your own

Hair gel: Instead of gel, mix noncarbonated or flat beer with water as a final rinse to control flyaway hair and keep it in place. Try a stiffly beaten egg white as a protein-enriching styling mousse. Simmer one tablespoon of flaxseeds in 1 cup of water until slightly thickened for a setting lotion. Substitute your regular hairspray with a spritz of lemon juice from a misting bottle to add resiliency, body, and highlights. Put your wax stick on the back burner and try blending 1 teaspoon of instant, dry milk (whole milk for normal to dry hair, skim for oily hair) with 1 cup water to create a wave. For homemade pomade, brew double-strength rosemary tea to preserve curls in damp weather (use only on darker hair colors).

Color Formulations, Perms, and Relaxers

These chemical treatments are designed to help change the color, texture, and structure of your hair. For best results, try both types of treatments in a salon under professional guidance; if performed incorrectly, the results can be disastrous. And don't attempt to create your own formulas. The risk of seriously damaging your hair isn't worth playing chemist.

make your own

Chamomile and Calendula Hair Lightener: The bright yellow of chamomile and calendula flowers resembles the sun and is bound to brighten your hair the same way. This temporary rinse lightens and brightens blond hair, increasing its softness and adding movement. Gentle highlights add texture and depth of color. Botanical formula: 4 cups water, 2 cups dried chamomile flowers, 2 cups dried calendula flowers, 1 tablespoon lemon juice, and 1 tablespoon lemon extract.

In a saucepan, bring water, chamomile, and calendula to a boil. Reduce heat, cover, and simmer for 45 minutes. Remove from heat, strain liquid into a bowl or pitcher, and stir in lemon juice and extract. When cool enough for application, stand in your shower and slowly pour the solution over your head, massaging it into your hair to cover all strands thoroughly. Cover hair with a plastic shower cap. Leave on for at least 40 minutes, then remove shower cap and rinse hair thoroughly with warm water. Use every other day for lasting effects.

make your own

Black Tea–Rosemary Rinse for Dark Brown Hair: Use the strong qualities of black teas and richly roasted coffees to add natural dark brown highlights to hair without damaging it. Tea and coffee, which are known to stain, are perfect for coloring brown hair. Rosemary is also an exceptional coloring agent for brown hair. Use the following recipe every other day on light to dark brown hair to add richness to brown hair of any shade. For a milder effect, use one less teaspoon of coffee and one less tea bag.

Botanical formula: 7 bags black tea or 2^1/$_2$ tablespoons loose tea, 2 tablespoons chopped oregano leaves, 2 tablespoons chopped rosemary leaves, 2 cups water, 1 tablespoon instant coffee, 1 tablespoon lemon extract. In a saucepan over medium heat, mix the tea, oregano, and rosemary with the water; steep for 45–50 minutes. Remove tea bags and filter out oregano, rosemary and loose tea if used. Place liquid in a small pitcher. Add coffee and lemon extract to liquid and stir until combined. Let cool, then while standing in your shower slowly pour the solution over your head, massaging it into your hair and scalp and covering all strands thoroughly. Cover hair with a plastic shower cap for 30 minutes. Remove shower cap and rinse hair thoroughly with warm water.

make your own

Oil Treatment: Weekly hot oil treatments can add luster and shine to the hair. Oils that most effectively penetrate the hair include olive oil, almond oil, avocado oil, safflower oil, and corn oil. Here's how to do it yourself: Heat $1/4$ cup of oil in a small saucepan over a very low flame until just warm. Remove from heat and let cool for about one minute. Massage warm oil into your hair. Cover hair with a plastic shower cap and then with a towel wrap. Leave on for 30 minutes, then rinse and shampoo as usual. Or, try this creative concoction from Philip B.:

Honey-Maple Hot Oil Treatment Botanical Formula:
1 teaspoon canola oil, 1 teaspoon margarine (softened), 1 tablespoon olive oil, 1 teaspoon coconut oil or extract, 1 teaspoon orange oil or extract, 1 tablespoon light sesame oil, 1 teaspoon macadamia nut oil, 1 teaspoon avocado oil, 1 teaspoon maple syrup, 1 teaspoon honey. Put all ingredients into a small saucepan, except for the syrup and honey. Heat over a very low flame until just warmed (about 2–3 minutes). Remove from heat. Cool for about 1 minute and add syrup and honey. Test with your finger to make sure it's not too hot to apply to scalp. Massage oil mixture into hair and then cover with a plastic shower cap. Leave on for 10 to 20 minutes. Remove shower cap and apply a mixture of equal parts shampoo and water and work into hair. Lather and rinse.

Chapter 3

The Kindest Cut

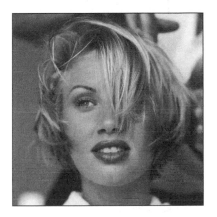

Cut to the Chase

Getting a new haircut isn't as simple as saying, "I want Jennifer Aniston's hair!" It may not be right for your face, your career, or your lifestyle. But thanks to today's high-tech styling tools, problem-specific products, and seriously skilled hairdressers, you can pretty much make any style you want work for you.

"It's important to know what you want to achieve and to communicate that to your hairdresser," says Oribe, consulting stylist to L'Oréal. "Look at pictures in magazines to decide what you like and stick with it. If you want to grow your hair out, don't let the hairdresser cut the length. If it needs maintenance during the grow-out period, find a hairdresser who will tell you how to maintain your style. The modern way of looking at hair is to think about what makes you feel great."

MYTH: Hair should be cut every three weeks.

FACT: Your hair needs to be cut on a regular basis to maintain healthy ends, style, and shape. However, the timing of cuts is based on individual growth rates and personal comfort level. There's no set time between cuts. And since hair grows at different rates seasonally, cutting times will differ according to the time of year.

The truth is these days you can have any hairstyle you want. If you love bangs and they fit your personality but don't necessarily jibe with the shape of your round face, the offbeat look you achieve is the individuality we're all searching for. And your hairdresser can help you choose the right products to make the look work for you—from color to texture changes to styling aids. If you have a conservative job and you want to look sexier for evening, your cut needs to be versatile; it has to be able to be blown out into something smooth or conservative for day or, with the right products, to be styled more wildly for night. If you work out in the middle of your work-day, you should have a style that can be pulled back and secured but can be easily reshaped into a look that makes others take you seriously at work. Layered hair can give you that versatility. According to Oribe, the biggest mistake you can make is to allow a stylist to push you into something that's not for you. "While it's important to stay realistic in what you want, if you find your hairdresser not willing to work with you, make sure you communicate your goals better," says Oribe. "Let your individuality dictate your look."

Choosing a Stylist

You may think finding a good hairstylist is like putting a $100 chip on black 17 on the roulette wheel. But you're wrong: Winning the bet is pure chance; finding the right stylist for you is pure science. So before you let just any old hairdresser start snipping, you might want to do some homework. Here is some stylist-searching advice from Joelle, senior stylist at Avon Salon and Spa, who says the most important thing is that you feel comfortable with your stylist.

- Ask people whose hair you like where they get it done and the name of the stylist who cuts it.

- Look at magazines to find out who did specific models' and celebrities' hair for specific events.

- Call the salon where that person works and schedule an appointment for a consultation with the stylist. Most salons offer complimentary consultations.

- When you arrive, interview the stylist. Start by introducing yourself, explaining who recommended the stylist to you, and ask how the stylist envisions your hair.

- Be direct. Specify your problems; discuss what you want your hair to look like, and how much time you have to spend to maintain that look in your daily routine. If you need to wash and go, tell the stylist your hair has to function that way. Not speaking up is the most common mistake women make.

- Keep in mind that one style may be great for your girlfriend's hair but might not work well for you.

- It's a good sign when a stylist asks a lot of specific questions to make an assessment about you as a person, what your capabilities are, how much time you have to spend on your hair, what type of look your profession requires. It's a bad sign if a hairdresser just wants to be creative and do your hair however he/she wants, if he/she dismisses your ideas and speaks to you in a condescending manner, or if the first thing he/she does is criticize your last stylist. A professional person who doesn't agree with your current style will simply offer advice on how to take it from there.

- Find out what the stylist's vision is for your hair, and if you feel uncertain about it, discuss your hesitations.

- Has he/she listened to you? Does he/she factor in what you said? All this is important in the hopes that this will be a long-lasting relationship, not just a one-shot deal.

- If you still don't know if the look is right for you, you are under no obligation to go ahead with the cut. Thank the stylist and let him/her know you'll think about it. Otherwise, you will end up getting a haircut, paying for it, and continuing the search for the right person at your own expense.

Giving a stylist free creative range is great if you're a wear-anything, do-anything kind of woman, adds Joelle, and if you're so confident that you'll love whatever he/she creates.

Taking Your Haircut(ter) Home

If you can't find the time to get to the salon for your routine trim, look for a pro who comes right to your door. New York City hairstylist Steven Shames is known as "the house-call hairdresser," traveling to women's homes to shear their locks. "You don't really know someone until you're in their home," says Shames. "It's easy for my clients because they can take a shower and wash their hair, then get their hair cut in the privacy of their own home. "It's very comfortable." Shames, who comes equipped with a plastic floor cover so you don't have to clean up shorn hair after he leaves, says seeing people's homes gives him a good idea of what they are all about, which helps him create a cut that suits their lifestyle. "Many people leave the salon and their hair looks fabulous, but when they try to do it themselves, they are completely lost," he says. "I'm very conscious of the fact that women have to do their hair themselves after I leave, so I tell them what they can do, which products they can use, and I explain what I'm doing to their hair throughout the cut. Seeing their hair for the first time is also indicative of what they can do on their own," explains Shames. "I always look at the front pieces because 99 percent of the time, the hair around the face is styled the way they want it and the way they feel comfortable with it."

How do you find a stylist who makes house calls in your town? If you live in an urban area you can often find them listed in the business section of the telephone book. They may also have websites, so search the Internet. Call salons—they may have cutters who are willing to travel. And word of mouth is good too. Many freelancers don't advertise in conventional ways, so asking friends and colleagues may turn up some good leads.

The Right Shape for Your Face

"The final result of the shape should always read sexy and modern with a bit of edge or originality," says veteran hairdresser John Sahag. "The right stylist can make any cut work for you by adapting it to your look. It's a

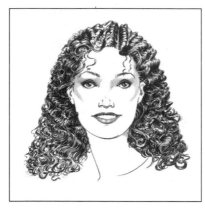

Oval faces look best in longer lengths, featuring face-framing layers that skim cheekbones and add width and make long faces appear shorter.

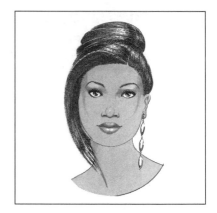

Round faces look best in styles that fall below the chin. Face-framing layers from the lips down remove weight from sides. Wispy, tapered ends de-emphasize roundness.

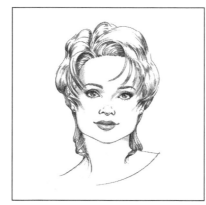

Square faces can carry off anything but one-length bobs. Short or long texturized ends and a long fringe graduating downward add height to the crown and balance out a square jaw.

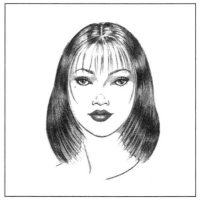

Heart-shaped faces look good in long, wavy layers that grace cheekbones and fall around the neck and take the emphasis off the chin. It is best to avoid blunt cuts, chunky bangs, or chopped layers, which will broaden the top half of the face.

visual art; the way you shape the whole thing makes a difference." Holding fast to the belief that straight lines are a thing of the past, Sahag's method is to continually chip into the texture to make it more intriguing. Some argue that in the struggle to match style to face structure, the old rules still apply.

Oval faces look best in longer lengths, featuring face-framing layers that skim cheekbones and add width; make a long face appear shorter with layers starting at the shoulder and bangs cut to eye level. Square faces can carry off anything but one-length bobs. Short or long texturized ends and a long fringe graduating downward add height to the crown and balance out a square jaw. Long hair layers starting at the jaw line lengthen the face. If you have a round face, stick to styles that fall below the chin. Face-framing layers from the lips down remove weight from sides, wispy and tapered ends de-emphasize roundness. For heart-shaped faces, try long, wavy layers that grace cheekbones and fall around the neck and take the emphasis off the chin; avoid blunt-cut lines, chunky bangs, or chopped layers that broaden the top half of the face. "What makes a cut modern is the feeling you capture in the end result, the uniqueness of the shape and how it's carved," adds Sahag. "It should look outstanding without looking outrageous. The shape should look like it belongs to you no matter what the length or texture, no matter whether you have short, medium-length, or long, curly, wavy, or straight hair."

Fixing Cut and Styling Mistakes

"We think it's the end of the world when we get a haircut we hate, when it's not working for us," says Mark Garrison of New York's Mark Garrison Salon. "But hair does grow, we're guaranteed of that. The best solution is to really do your homework, find the right stylist for what you want to do, discuss the details of the cut over and over, and don't be afraid that you're being neurotic about what it will look like or how to manage it. Remember, what you may think is a bad haircut may be a cut you just never learned how to style, so make sure your stylist shows you how to do it yourself." Garrison says he always shows his clients how to manage their hair naturally, so they know that's an option. If you still can't seem to get the style right, feel free to call the salon back and ask for help.

Hair is a medium that's forever changing and growing, and we are constantly readjusting, rebalancing, and reproportioning our hair to compensate. "A great cut that's grown out isn't flattering anymore," says Garrison. "There are three factors involved: whether or not the cut is shaped to flatter your bone structure, whether you're trying to protect your hair's natural texture, and whether the cut fits into your lifestyle. You can have a bad haircut if any one of these factors is not jibing." It's not a good sign if you have to work at it too much. Garrison suggests some solutions to some of the most common "bad haircut" problems: If there's too much volume on the sides, have your stylist layer or angle the sides to reduce volume or pick up the length in back to balance out the sides. If your bangs have been cut too short or straight across the forehead, grow them out, then soften them with layers with a razor or texturizing scissors or cut into the tips with regular scissors. If curly hair is cut too short, it will end up looking like a ball around your face. To get a straighter, sleeker style, you may want to leave longer bangs in a bit of an angle, so a piece can dangle around the cheekbone, and keep the length long enough so that it stays flat on the sides or angles to correspond with your cheekbones and with the width of your face. Angling and layering the sides can lift hair up and away from cheekbones and reduce the pyramid effect. Keep in mind that what's hot on the runway isn't always right for you. The one-length, off-the-shoulder bob, which caused a stir throughout the fashion world, actually makes hair fall in a pyramid shape with lots of weight around the bottom and most women can't handle it. The best remedy for bad haircuts? According to Garrison, it's hair accessories. "Barrettes or clips hold back bangs that aren't cut correctly. Headbands, combs, and scarves disguise bad cuts and dress them up at the same time."

Styling Without Damaging

Now that you know how to rectify a bad cut, what can you do on a regular basis to avoid serious damage to your hair? Carmine Minardi identifies two kinds of damage: First, there is desirable damage, which happens when we intentionally want to break down the cuticle, as in relaxing, perming, or coloring hair from dark to light. Second, there is undesirable damage, which can occur from chemical processing such as perms, bleach, chemical relaxers, or color that's not administered correctly or is overused. It can also stem from cutting and styling techniques such as razor cutting or flat-ironing.

"Slicing hair tips on an angle gives hair good texture but, if you overdo it, you will make hair appear frizzy and dry. It may not really be in bad condition, but it will present your hair in poor condition. The heat from flat irons can also cause damage; they should only be used for three to four seconds per section of hair. The objective is to press hair down and slide it through the iron without holding it for an extended period of time. In addition, tremendous amounts of moisture will make hair appear as though it's dried out, deadened, and lifeless." Minardi adds that women with highlighted, high-lifted, and highly processed hair should be cautious about using finishing sprays that contain a lot of alcohol or products that contain liquid plastics, like hair thickeners or certain gels. "They make hair extremely porous and can leave it feeling crunchy to the touch when it dries." Women shouldn't be overly concerned with damage from in-salon treatments, which are performed by experts who are experienced at using these

> **Set Yourself Free: How to Escape When Your Brush Gets Caught in Your Hair**
>
> The last thing you want to do is wear your hairbrush as an accessory. Before you panic and run aimlessly down the street to the nearest salon, follow this advice: Pulling at the brush to try to get it out will only tangle your hair further. Instead, use your opposite hand to gently pull as much hair as possible out of the brush in separate sections. Eventually, you will have removed enough so that the brush can be freed easily.

Score! Get Your Hair Done By a Pro—(For Very Little Dough)

Many major salons and beauty schools hold regular training sessions to help educate their stylists, colorists, and students. You could be a model and get your hair done for a great rate! "We focus on the fundamentals of hair cutting and coloring," says Nikki An-Levy, stylist/educator for Bumble and Bumble hair salon in New York City. "When someone comes to work here as an assistant, they need to start off learning different techniques first with scissors and then with razors, which are used more often to create movement and shape. We work in levels, from basic scissor cuts to longer layers, to bobs, to short- haired scissor cuts. It's all about understanding the technique, the shape of the head, and how each hair texture will react."

The salon holds classes every Monday, and the assistants who are training that night are responsible for getting women to volunteer. As if they have to twist their arms! "The hardest part is finding the right model for the haircut we need to perfect. We need women who are willing to try it and have fun with it." Remember, training cuts will be significantly cheaper than regular salon cuts, so if you are on a budget, it may be a great way to get a fabulous cut or color job. Think you're the perfect candidate for a salon training-night cut?

Here's what to do:
DO call your local salon to find out if they have a training program. If they do, volunteer your services. You can also check out beauty schools—they also offer times when students cut volunteers' hair—and sometimes the cuts are free!

DON'T be nervous about trying something fun and different. Now's your chance to see how the latest 'do will look on you.

DO talk to the cutter before he or she starts to make sure you know what kind of cut they will be doing. Hair grows back—but not overnight. So, be sure you know what you will be getting.

products. But when it comes to styling tools you use at home, only you can control the amount of damage you subject your hair to.

Dry Ideas

If you think you can only get a good, professional-looking cut if your hair is wet, think again. Dry cuts have been gaining in popularity in recent years, and there's good reason for it.

"For years, people have been getting their hair washed and their hairdresser would cut it wet. I was one of first people to cut hair dry," says Edward Tricomi, co-owner and stylist of the Warren Tricomi Salon in New York City. "When I was on set working for the magazines, I would wash, cut, and blow-dry the hair, and if I didn't like it I would rethink the whole idea of the style and recut the hair. I always felt that when hair was dry, I could see what it was doing better."

Tricomi, who has been dry-cutting the hair of celebs such as Mick Jagger and Barbra Streisand for twenty-six years, swears by the method. "I cut multilevels in the hair," he explains. "I use thinning shears to create sublevels, and I use a pair of scissors like a pencil to sketch through the haircut." Tricomi says he owes his great coordination to his musical roots (he used to play the drums). "I pick up the hair and let it fly," he says. "As it's flying, I catch it in various places with a scissor, flickering through it in a random yet calculated manner. In nature, things grow at random and have many dimensions to them, and that's how I cut hair."

Styling with Color and Highlights

"Hair color has become an integral part of a haircut," says Beth Minardi, who co-owns the Minardi hair salon in New York City with her husband, Carmine. "If someone has wonderful hair that's cut in varying layers and is all one color, you won't see the layers well. Coloring sections of the hair allows the nuance of light and dark so you can see the shape of the cut." Minardi also uses color as an accenting tool. She explains that women with a broad jaw can have lighter sections placed at the temples to draw attention to the forehead instead. "Color helps accent parts of the cut to give the appearance of more texture and body and to play up skin tone," says Minardi. She points out that the wrong color can make hair look bushier, but a subtle shade-on-shade can make hair look smoother. Should you have your hair cut or colored first? "For a trim, it doesn't matter," she says, "but for a big change like a whole new shape, we color it first so it's easy to see where it will fall."

Bridal Style

"The biggest mistake brides make is listening to advice from too many different people," says Chuck Jones, bridal director of Elizabeth Arden Salon in New York City, who has a special formula for helping brides decide how to wear their hair. Here are the steps he takes to help women choose the style for the most perfect day of their life:

1. "The sooner I meet with a bride the better," says Jones, "so we can work toward the right cut and color for the wedding day."

2. "Every time a girl goes out to a party or special event during the time we are working together," says Jones, "I do her hair a different way so she has a chance to try out several different styles and decide which one she likes best and feels most comfortable in."

3. "Most women have three fittings for their dress," says Jones. "I do their hair differently for each of the fittings so they can see which hair style best complements their dress.

4. "The biggest debate is whether a bride should wear her hair up or down," says Jones. "I always recommend a bride wear her

hair up so it's out of the way, unless she wants to wear it down because she always wears it down."

5. "If you wear your hair up, you need to make sure the style will hold," says Jones. "Keep pins and hair spray in the bridal room for necessary touch-ups. If you wear it down, you want to ensure that you don't have stringy hair by the end of the night. Remember, you'll be dancing a lot and you'll be kissing and hugging people all day."

6. "I'm here to guide brides on hairstyles and help them save money on veils and headpieces," says Jones. "For example, some bridal shops try to sell a particular headpiece with a particular dress and tell brides that they are sold together. But you can choose a different headpiece if you like another one better."

7. "I bring a camera and take a picture of each bride in her dress with her hair done so she can compare it to previous fittings and decide which image she likes best," says Jones, who can tailor a hairstyle for a morning or evening event. "All that's left of the big day after it's over is the pictures and the video," says Jones. "I want the bride to look back ten years from now and say, 'I looked lovely!' not 'Who talked me into that?'"

Razor Rules

"In the past, I've found mild hesitation in clients as well as stylists when it comes to using a razor to cut hair," says Jason Low, stylist at Peter Coppola in New York City. "Maybe they had a bad experience at one time or another. But attitudes have changed because razor-cutting is currently more in vogue and the technique has been refined." Low, who trained in London, says he determines what kinds of tools to use depending on the shape he wants to achieve and the texture of his client's hair. "A razor is great on certain textures but murder on others," he says. "If razor-cutting isn't appropriate for a client's hair texture, it won't work." The best candidates are women with shorter shapes as well as Asian hair or thinner, finer hair.

In addition, anyone who is willing to go shorter can really benefit. Finally, anyone who's had a bad hair cut will love it. "The razor is very forgiving to cuts gone bad," says Low. Those who should avoid the technique: women with incredibly highlighted hair or very, very curly hair. "Using a razor," he explains, "is like using one side of a pair of scissors and sliding through the hair instead of chopping it up. It gives hair a seamless edge by cutting hair on an angle instead of straight down." Some stylists think the razor is more sculpting. "It's very systematic; there's more architecture involved," says Low. "Using a razor makes the cut incredibly stick-straight and makes the hair flow without any lines or steps whatsoever.

"When the cut is complete, you can see that the shape looks more fluid and everything blends nicely." The bottom line: "As long as the stylist knows what he/she is doing, the result is so much more fine-tuned and tailored," says Low. "It can take the bulk out of certain shapes and lessen the weight while keeping everything in proportion."

Dread Heads

Dreads are not a temporary, carefree hairstyle. The technique of tightly knotting (not braiding!) your hair takes a while to achieve and, once you have gotten the dreads tight, they are difficult, if not downright impossible, to undo. But dreadlocks aren't permanent either. If you do have well-established dreads, you will most likely have to cut them to about three inches if you want to move on to a new style. That means the decision to dread your hair should not be taken lightly.

It's better to start your dreads when your hair is fairly long. However, you can start the process even if your hair is only three inches long. Any shorter and it will be pretty difficult to get the right twist going.

Start with small sections of hair (have a friend help you with the back) and start twisting and waxing with a product like Dread Head wax. Until your dreadlocks "mature" you'll need to play with them a lot. The more you twist and tangle the roots and the ends the faster they will grow into tight, healthy, and knotty dreads. Creating dreadlocks is a very interactive experience! You will really get to know your hair along the way.

You'll need to comb and wax your dreads pretty regularly to keep them tightened and fresh-looking. If your hair is short, wearing rubber bands at the root and tip of the dread will hold the hair secure, giving it time to tighten. If you have a lot of hair, dreading is easier. But if you have thick strands of hair, it will take longer since it's harder to get it to stay in knots. Dread Head wax will help dread any type of hair. Perming thick hair or leaving it in braids for a day or two before will make it dread much easier. If your hair is really thin or if you don't have that much of it, dreads can make your hair appear fuller and thicker.

Dreadlocked hair needs regular washing. The best way to keep your locks clean is by thoroughly wetting your hair and then gently working the soap in and then squeezing and rinsing hair repeatedly to get all the soap out. Don't pull your dreads when they are soapy! This will loosen your locks, exactly the opposite of what you want to happen. Rinsing is important too—you don't want any residue left behind because that can affect the tightness of your locks. Clean, residue-free hair locks up faster than dirty or oily hair. Choosing the right shampoo, one that's not heavily perfumed or filled with extra conditioners and moisturizers, is also essential. Natural shampoos make rinsing easier. When you are just starting to dread, or if you feel your locks aren't tight enough to withstand a straight under-the-shower shampoo, try stretching a clean panty hose leg over your hair. Washing the dreads through the fine nylon mesh will prevent hair from coming loose.

To brush your dreads, use a soft bristle brush and start from the bottom, gently working your way up. Avoid tugging or aggressive brushing, as this could weaken the locks and break individual hairs. To keep dreads in place as you sleep, gently tie up your hair with a soft cotton band. Never go to bed with your hair wet.

If, after a week, you decide that you want to go back to your old style, don't worry. A hot shower and lots of conditioner will melt the wax and help untangle the knots. It may take some time, but be patient and gentle.

Hairstylist Alberto Guzman, who creates dreads for music-industry celebs, offers some insider's tips on creating a dreaded style:

- Weave or twist synthetic dreadlocks in different colors (from blond to blue!) into your hair for a pop of color and texture.

- Twist and blow-dry dreads individually. Then pull them back and tie them into a ponytail at the crown for an elegant, classic look.

- Attach a hairpiece with dreadlocks onto your head for a temporary dread. Use hair and bobby pins to lock it into place so you can dance without fear of losing it.

Back to Business: Hair and Work

In the same way you have to choose your clothes to suit your job, you have to wear your hair to complement your profession. Female athletes often cut their hair into a short bob to keep it off their face. Other active women with long hair may braid it, partially to make a fashion statement and partially to keep it in place. Tennis champs Venus and Serena Williams come to mind in this regard. Women in corporate America often opt for more conservative styles and used to run the risk of having "hard hair," or "helmet head." We still see product-laden styles now and then, but these days, luckily, more hair and less 'do seems to be the trend. Soft, classic hair that matches your hair type really is the best bet if you are unsure of what to do stylewise. One thing is certain: No matter what career you choose, the way you wear your hair can have an effect on your success and the way you feel at work. Here, three women share their on-the-job hair rules:

✦

Katy, executive chef:

"The most important thing is that the stylist leaves enough length so I can pull it back. And I don't wear bangs anymore. I try to keep all of the hair off my face as much as possible. I'll put it in a shoulder-length ponytail or a twist. In addition, I like my hair to smell nice, so I make sure I take good care of it. The kitchen doesn't do that much damage. It doesn't make your hair smell because there are usually pretty good commercial ventilation systems and there are fans to suck up the smoke. It can get greasy though; most of the line cooks go home after their shifts and take a shower immediately. You tend to sweat a lot more in the kitchen too (because it's so hot!), so it helps if you keep your hair up and off your neck.

"The only sacrifice I think I've made in cutting my hair because of my profession is to avoid getting layers, since they fall in your face more. If I didn't have my job, I would choose to have layers. Hair falls better when you can do that. I also think a lot of female chefs go short with their hair. I have such a long neck that if I don't have length, my hairstyle accentuates the length of my neck."

✦

Cindy, veterinarian:

"As a veterinarian, I work around animals all day long, so I try to keep my hair long so I can pull it back if I lean over a dog or cat to examine them and it gets in the way. If your hair touches the animal, you can run the risk of fungus or parasites, which can transfer to your hair and scalp. In addition, if your hair touches an animal that has ringworm and you touch your hand to your hair, you can contaminate other animals. When you're in surgery, certain sterile procedures require that we wear our hair up so we don't dip it into anything. Still, anything can happen. I'm just glad I don't work for a large-animal vet; some of the smallest procedures on large animals can be very smelly, even after several days of showers and baths! For those vets, their hair smells like a barn—all the time."

✦

Pam, executive assistant:

"Put-together, polished, stylish yet conservative is the image my boss likes his employees to convey. Looking good on my job is important because my boss deals with an older, more conservative crowd and he wants me to look professional. My boss responds better to me when I'm more put-together. I wear my hair back in a ponytail at work, as do a lot of women; it's easier to work that way, without having it fall in your face. It also helps exude a professional image, not a sexy one. Curly, wild hair is a little more extreme. In fact, most of the women I work with have straighter hair.

"When I go to the salon, I want the latest style but not something too trendy and too crazy. I've been at my job for ten years now, so I know what I can and can't wear. I try to have a different image at work than when I go out socially. Many times, if I'm planning on going out after work, I change my clothes and let my hair down—literally. There is a girl in my office who sometimes wears cornrows. My boss won't tell her not to wear them, but I can tell it bothers him. That's more of a fun way to wear your hair, not a professional way.

"When I was younger, I would take more risks with my hair. The day before a 'milestone' birthday, I got a little crazy and got a perm. I had a party on a boat and by the end of the trip it looked like I had just stuck my hand in an electric socket. I would never do anything that crazy now when I have to be at work the next day. Although, over the years I have seen more progressive style changes in the way executive assistants can dress and wear their hair."

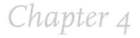

Hair Treatments

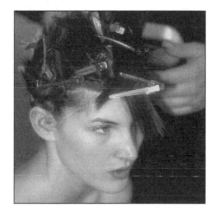

Take a cue from celebrities who continuously change their hair color for film roles and public appearances. Gwyneth Paltrow, Winona Ryder, Angelina Jolie, Renee Russo, and supermodel Linda Evangelista all know how much fun a new shade can be. After all, changing your color, adding a few highlights, curling, relaxing, or wearing your hair in braids can really add life to your hair and lift your mood. Most of these treatments involve chemical processes that can make your hair look amazing, but they can also cause major damage if used incorrectly. So follow these tips on how to have the look you love without sacrificing your locks.

Get Color Courageous

Letting people know you color your hair used to be almost as much of a taboo as talking about your sex life. Women only colored their hair if they wanted to completely change the color, or if they wanted to cover their gray. In the 21st century, however, with more than 50 percent of women in the United States coloring their hair, it's not only acceptable, it's a sign of being fashion forward and up with the trends. What's more, it's easy to do and less damaging to your hair than it was a couple of decades ago.

Finding a professional colorist is the key to soft, richly hued hair. Those colorists who have honed their skills are being well rewarded financially and raised to celebrity status. Therefore appointments often fill up months in advance. "A reputable colorist provides a very detailed consultation, taking the time to explain the techniques involved in the process," says Bob Siebert, national director of education for Hans Schwarzkopf Professional. "A good colorist will also give you a road map for maintenance, explaining what you can do to maintain your color at home and make it last until you come in for your next visit, about five to six weeks later."

It's best to color your hair at a salon where experts use high-quality color and are experienced enough to know how to do it right—especially if you want a major change. For smaller jobs, like touching up your roots or covering gray, you can probably pull it off at home by reading the directions that come with the product.

Color Maintenance

Since bleach and dyes can dry out hair and damage the cuticle, color-processed hair needs a little extra TLC. Avoid shampoos that contain Castille soaps or oil or glycerin, which may fade the color, or clarifying shampoos, which may strip the color. Your best bet is to choose a shampoo with extra conditioning properties. Companies such as Thermasilk, Aveda, Revlon, Vidal Sassoon, and Artec offer these specialized formulas, and more and more color-maintenance lines are popping up regularly.

Permanent hair color is the most popular because it lasts the longest, delivers all-over, even color, and creates the most dramatic change. How it works: In a single process, peroxide and ammonia are mixed. "The ammonia opens up the cuticle and allows the pigment to penetrate into the cortex where the natural pigment is," says Siebert. "The melanin in your hair is oxidized and loses its natural color." According to Siebert, this single process procedure is ideal for women who want to cover gray or lighten their hair a couple of shades from their natural color. Permanent color, however, is the most damaging to your hair, and can make it look flat and unnatural, requiring frequent touchups. Although the formulations vary in potency, most ammonia-containing brands dry out hair and cause it to frizz.

"Double processing—the most aggressive form of coloring hair— requires two steps," explains Siebert. "First, hair is pre-lightened with lightening powder or bleach, then the color or highlights are applied afterward."

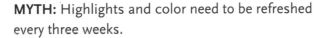

MYTH: Highlights and color need to be refreshed every three weeks.

FACT: Hair grows at different rates, and this affects how long color and highlights last. The color itself, and its difference from hair's natural shade, plays a part in how frequently it needs revitalizing. Some women find they need roots "done" every two weeks; some can go a month.

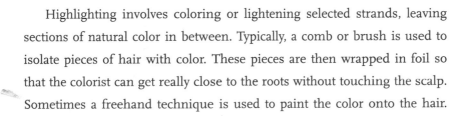

Highlighting involves coloring or lightening selected strands, leaving sections of natural color in between. Typically, a comb or brush is used to isolate pieces of hair with color. These pieces are then wrapped in foil so that the colorist can get really close to the roots without touching the scalp. Sometimes a freehand technique is used to paint the color onto the hair.

Salon Shades vs. Home Hues

"Everything from cell phones to cars to communication has taken an edge toward fashion. Hair color is the opposite; we have always had the artistic edge, but now we have the technology behind it," says Deborah Gavin, a stylist and colorist at High Tech salon in Philadelphia. "For many women, hair color is an important expression of who they are and how they want the world to see them." Here, she shares her top reasons for having hair professionally colored:

1. Professional color is more advanced and more durable.

2. With professional color, you're not just paying for the hair color itself, but also for a colorist's technical and application skills.

3. You are also getting the colorist's ability to choose the right shade for your skin tone. When you do it yourself at home, what you see on the box isn't exactly what you end up with.

4. "Most women aren't skilled enough to apply their own color, especially because the angle is difficult. The only time it works is when you get lucky with it. Otherwise, it can look uneven and may deliver the message that you don't care as much about how you look," she says.

5. Professional hair color can be strategically placed. "Techniques for applying hair color are constantly evolving. Transformation color, one such method, involves using different shades of the same color on different sections of hair, depending on how you part your hair. "You can part your hair on one side and have the color there done in a natural shade of red, which may appear more conservative for work. Then, you can part your hair on the other side and color that section with a brighter shade for post-office hours."

6. Some experts argue that at-home brands contain lesser percentages of color so that you need to buy more to achieve the color you desire. Others say it is dangerous for women to do their own color because most at-home versions come in shampoo form and, except for the first application, you really just need to touch up the roots. It is more damaging to shampoo over previously colored hair.

"Highlighting and lowlighting give hair more dimension," says Siebert. "Highlights brighten hair by adding light, while lowlights use darker tones to add depth to the hair." The end result is a beautiful, subtly brighter head of hair, but the time-consuming process means you may not get to see it until you've been worked on for a couple of hours.

"Long-lasting semipermanent or demipermanent color is the quickest-growing color segment in the market for professional and retail color," explains Siebert. "The benefit is that in most cases they are ammonia-free, so they are a little more gentle on hair. This is a great way for clients to try on color if they're not ready to make a commitment; they fade out in 15 to 30 shampoos." Semipermanent color penetrates the hair shaft and stains the cuticle, so it isn't as dense as permanent color and it's less noticeable when it fades. Semipermanent color can be used on permed hair and is applied in liquid, gel, or aerosol form. Demipermanent color is used to enhance your natural color and cover 75 percent of gray. But since it only deposits color without lifting your hair's natural pigment, it won't lighten your hair. So while that means you won't have roots to contend with, it will probably fade within six weeks. If you have a fear of commitment, try a temporary color or a rinse, which washes out in three to seven shampoos. "These are made of 100 percent preoxidized pigments that are not mixed with developer or peroxide," explains Siebert. "They stain the outer layer of hair, then wash away." Often made of a vegetable dye base, temporary colors are applied directly from the tube or bottle in the form of a rinse, gel, mousse, or spray. Funkier versions, such as hair mascara, are now available on the market, and can be fun for a night when you dare to go bold with your hair color.

Natural hair color is ideal for women who are allergic to aniline, a colorless liquid obtained from coal tar from which many hair colors and dyes are made. Reactions to aniline include itchy red patches and welts on the scalp. Natural colors stain the hair instead of dyeing it and don't penetrate the hair shaft. While several hair color companies sell natural, commercial hair color, only pure Egyptian henna is truly organic. Made from the leaves of the *lawsonia inermis* plant, henna colors by coating the hair shaft and staining the cuticle. The color is unpredictable and hard to control and not for women with permed hair, since it can clash with the perming chemicals and cause discoloration. If you're using henna at home, be sure to wear gloves so you don't stain your hands.

In the 1960s, a hair technique called tipping was extremely popular. Using this method, bleach is applied only to the ends of the hair to make them a lighter shade than the rest of the head. Today, this method is often done using color instead of bleach. "Bleaching can be used in two different ways," adds Amanda George, a colorist at Prive salon in Los Angeles, "for an overall blond effect à la Marilyn Monroe, or as a double-blonding process by lifting hair all over then bringing it up a tone to beige blond or platinum blond. When you color hair blond, there's a limit to how light you can go, because it depends on how dark your hair is to begin with. If someone wants a really light shade of blond, pre-lighten with bleach, then add color. For a softer, honey blond, skip the bleach and use tint plus highlights to get the right shade." At-home color is premixed and geared to cover a more generic range of shades, as opposed to salon color, which is individually mixed for you. Look for low-ammonia or low-peroxide products, which are gentler on your hair.

Which Coloring Technique Is Right for You?

Aside from the basic highlighting and lowlighting, Colin Lively, hair color director for Elizabeth Arden Red Door salon in New York City, helps us sort out the hair color methods you can choose from. Now, you'll be able to follow all that colorist lingo without feeling in the dark.

Foiling: This technique achieves exact placement of color. Specific strands of hair are selected to receive the color. The color in the foil doesn't touch any strands of hair outside the foil. The object is to create precise, multi-dimensional hair color. The end result: a very subtle look. Instead of foil, some colorists use plastic wrap or wax paper because they believe some foils, when interacting with certain hair colors, can create a chemical reaction on the hair that will end up looking brassy and may be damaging to the hair.

Hand-Painting: Hand-painting, which is done with a brush, strives for a diffused look. However, the residue from the painted areas is likely to bleed onto unpainted strands. Depending on your desired effect, this may be okay. But generally speaking, hand-painting or free-painting techniques are always more obvious than foiling.

Baliage: A roll of cotton is set near the base of the hair at the scalp. Hair color is applied to alternate sections of hair, and hair with hair color is placed across the cotton so that it arches as it comes off the scalp. The cotton prevents colored hair from touching hair that's not meant to be colored.

Frosting: This method is not as commonly used as it once was. It involves using a frosting cap (similar to a shower cap with holes in it). The cap is placed on the head and, using an instrument like a crochet hook, bits of hair are pulled through the holes in the cap. Hair color is applied to the top of the cap so that only selective strands are colored. The hair inside the cap will be protected. The result is multidimensional.

Choose a hair color kit that contains conditioning formulas that bind to the hair shaft and add moisture and shine. The dangerous thing about applying at-home color is that it's easy to overlap your products. "The goal is to put color on new hair and use a different product on the ends than on the roots. If you double-apply product on hair that's already been colored or permed, you can cause serious damage and breakage," says Sibert.

"Looking at the shelves can be overwhelming," says Julia Youssef, director of the technical center for L'Oréal. "It's important to know your hair type and be able to identify your hair color the way it is at the present time. Look at the color chart on the box, and try to determine if your color is close to the swatch on the box. If it is, you will get the result that is promised. If the color of your hair isn't identified on the box, that shade isn't good for you."

Once you are able to determine your initial hair color, know what you want. "You have to be able to say, 'I'm medium brown and I want to be a fiery redhead' or 'I'm dark blond and I want to be a light blond,' or 'I want to cover gray or add a bit of highlights to my medium brown hair,'" says Youssef.

"When determining their natural hair color, most people see their hair darker than it is," adds Sandy St. Roi, senior manager of product evaluation for Clairol. "Women with medium brown hair always say they have dark brown hair, women with medium blond hair often call it dark blond. It's vision lighting contrast. If you determine your natural hair too dark, you will choose the wrong indicator on the box." Roi suggests thinking of your natural shade as one level lighter than what you think it is and selecting hair color that's within two shades of your natural level. "If you're dark blond, light blond is a good selection but don't go to the lightest blond," she says. Once you have determined your needs, choose the box that appeals to you the most and promises to take care of them. "If you want to cover a full head of gray, look for 100 percent coverage of gray," suggests Youssef. "If the box says the color will gently chase away first grays, it's not going to give you maximum gray coverage. If it says it gently boosts and brightens natural highlights, it won't give you a drastic fashion change." It's also important to understand the type of color you are using, which is clearly marked on all at-home color boxes. Level three designates permanent hair color, designed to lighten or darken your shade and cover gray. Level two means semi- or demipermanent, or tone on tone, which is usually non-ammonia formula designed to enhance your current tone before it shampoos out within 28 shampoos. Level one, which isn't as popular anymore, is a rinse or temporary color. Common mistakes to watch out for: "If you choose a hair color according to the visual on the box because you think it looks beautiful instead of really acknowledging your own hair color and what you want to achieve, you won't get the color you're looking for," says Youssef. "If you don't leave the color on long enough because you don't want it to get too dark, you won't let it process correctly or completely and it won't look even. It's like taking a cake out of the oven before it's baked." L'Oréal's automatic shut-off feature means that if the recommended time is 20–25 minutes and you leave it on for 35 minutes, you won't have a problem. Youssef also advises that if you're doing a touch-up, do the roots first instead of all-over color to give the roots a 15-minute head start.

If you're doing your hair yourself, price is obviously a factor. "Most hair color costs ten dollars or less per box," says Roi. One box usually means one application, but, according to Roi, what you should realize is that if your hair is below shoulder length, or if you are trying it for the first time and are likely to make mistakes, you may need two boxes. Clairol's hair colors also include a patch test, which should be done prior to coloring hair to determine whether or not you are allergic to the color. They usually involve mixing a capful of color and developer, applying it to the inside of your elbow, and leaving it on for 48 hours to see your reaction.

"It's important to color at least a week before a special event to get the look you want to achieve," says Roi. At www.clairol.com, you can upload your picture and try on different colors. There are 590 shades and 159 hair-styles to choose from. Roi also advises current color users who want to make a major change—such as if you've been coloring your hair red and want to be a blonde—to refer to the company's 800 number, since it's a more complicated process. Experts can advise on removing the red tint before applying the new blond color and offer free personalized consultations to help you use the color correctly.

Companies like L'Oréal have been perfecting their home hair color systems for years with drip-free applicators, salon-quality gloves, fresh scents, and "color cues," in addition to information designed to help you choose the shade that's right for you. And in an attempt to offer women more intense, light-reflecting color, they have created illuminating and innovative new formulas that enhance color, make hair shine, and leave it looking natural. Other companies such as Schwarzkopf, which launched a new hair color with vitamin C, are going all out to protect against color fad-

make your own

Homemade hair dyes: The hulls of black walnuts, which are sold in health food stores, can be pressed to produce a juice that dyes hair dark brown. Wear rubber gloves when applying because it stains skin, too. For a rich hue, combine 1 cup walnut juice, 1 tablespoon ethyl alcohol, and 1 tablespoon each of ground cinnamon and cloves in a screw-top jar. Let stand for a week, shaking daily, then strain through a cloth-lined sieve and add 1 teaspoon salt. Homemade hennas are a bit easier to concoct. To brighten dark hair, try regular-strength brewed chamomile tea; rosemary and sage teas brighten as ▶

▶ they add glimmer. Leave on for a half hour, and then
rinse with warm water. To liven light hair, or add a reddish
shimmer to blond or light brown hair, try a final rinse
of green pekoe tea. Or, combine 1 cup water with $\frac{1}{2}$ cup
strained lemon juice to bring a touch of sunshine to
light hair.

ing. If you've tried making your own hair color, you've got too much time on your hands. It's a tricky process that shouldn't be messed with. But if you insist, try these tips for a cool new hue.

Of course, there's always the chance you might make a mistake. In that event, go to a pro. "Correcting color is one of the most rewarding things to execute," says Siebert, who is accustomed to typically working with hair that's been through many processes, and is regularly faced with the challenge of trying to make it look natural. "We try to create a uniform color result," he says. "We analyze each different area of hair and determine what needs to be done, whether it's lightening, overlightening, or pre-pigment. It's not as simple as applying one color on the whole thing and fixing it. We have to take into consideration the quality and strength of the hair. Our objective is to take clients to their most natural, even color with the least amount of damage."

Permanent Arrest

Perming is a chemical process that breaks the bonds in the hair's structure and reestablishes them in the shape of curls. When the process was first introduced to the general public more than seventy years ago, it was a dream come true for straight-haired women bored with their stick-straight locks and tired of all the effort it took to make their hair look a little livelier. Then, twenty years ago, body waves came on the scene, a milder form of the perm, which was created to add lift and body to thin, flat hair. "Perms aren't as popular now as they used to be," says Carmine Minardi of New York's Minardi Salon. "They used to make hair appear thicker or fatter. But hair color, highlights, and bleach all have an alkaline base, and this fattens the hair shaft. By coloring the hair shaft, you get a two-for-one deal, both color and body." Minardi warns that perms on top of color may be too much for your hair to handle. "Not all perms work well with color, so stay away from perms if you're using bleach or color. Use curling irons or other styling tools instead." Any perm veteran will wrinkle up her nose at the mere mention of the word perm—a term that is sure to conjure up smells of the intense perming solution that was used in the process in the old days when nitric acid and heat were used to wave hair. These days, perming formulas are more pleasantly scented and less harsh on your hair. In addition, stylists can use them to control the area of hair they want to perm and the softness of the curl. "It's about changing the bonds you were born with," says Minardi. "These disulfonic bonds are arranged like the rungs of a ladder in the hair shaft. Hair is wrapped around a curling rod, using a small rod for a tight curl or a larger rod for a looser curl. Ammonia or the sulfur-based chemical thioglycolate is applied to break the bonds of the hair and relax it, then a neutralizer is used to reattach the bonds in a new configuration and harden that new formation to create the curl."

Gentler perming solutions from companies like Zotos, Helene Curtis, and Senscience can be found in salons where they are used by experts who have mastered the application of these potent formulas. If you insist on administering your perm yourself, choose a solution that's thioglycolate-free and contains conditioner to soften hair.

At-home perms may save you a few bucks but can be tricky to choose and to self-administer. "In choosing an at-home perm, we want women to think about what they're doing to their hair, what they have done to their hair before, and what they want to accomplish now," says Adrienne Kent, marketing assistant for Colomer USA, the makers of Great Feeling, Equave, and Sensor perms in the Roux collection. "Go to a beauty supply store, look at the perm boxes, read the directions, then go home and call the 800 number on the box and ask all of your questions before you do it. Seek as much professional advice as you can before you do it to help achieve a better end result." Kent says it's also a good idea to get a consultation at a salon before doing it yourself.

Once you decide to take the plunge, follow the instructions carefully. After all, Roux perming

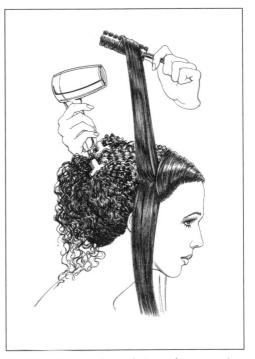

Straightening or relaxing hair can be a complex procedure, best undertaken by professionals.

instructions are always bi- or trilingual, with explanations in English, Spanish, and French to make sure you really understand what you're doing. "Do a strand test, follow the diagrams, which show you how to mix the solution, apply it, and roll your hair. Carefully monitor the timing suggested in the instructions, and read about what to do if you feel a tingling or burning sensation, so that you're prepared to handle it," says Kent.

Why all the caution? "Overprocessing is the biggest mistake," says Kent. "Some women tend to allow the perm to stay on too long or use the perming solution when they shouldn't because their hair has already been through a lot or is overprocessed." The bottom line: Know what your hair has been through and where you are taking it. "Perms last until the entire length of your hair grows out or until you cut it," says Oscar Bond, owner,

Oscar Bond salon in New York City. "You don't have to do anything to maintain your perm, but you should make an effort to maintain the condition of your hair by using extra conditioning treatments on a regular basis." Bond advises cutting off permed hair before getting a new perm or introducing your hair to other chemical processes.

Just Relax

Like perming, relaxing involves breaking the hair's natural bonds to eliminate any wave or curl. But instead of restructuring the bonds into a curlier configuration, the curls are loosened and the hair becomes stick-straight. Relaxing is popular among African-American women whose hair is most naturally curly.

Thinking of relaxing your hair yourself? Think again. "Relaxing your hair involves serious chemicals, and if you try it at home you can get severely burned," warns Valerie Estrada, master stylist, Allure Day Spa and Hair Salon in New York. "When using a relaxer, it's also possible to seriously damage your hair. You can miss pieces because you're not familiar with the proper technique, and if your hair is overporous and overly processed, it may break off." Estrada suggests going to a stylist who knows the history of your hair and can decide which product is best for you. Cream relaxers are often used on coarse hair because they totally relax the cuticle so that it's easier to blow out or flat iron. They make unruly hair easier to manage and help your newly straightened hair last longer. How it works: A cream or oil is applied to your scalp for protection, then chemicals are worked into your dry hair one section at a time. The hair will process until it's as straight as you want, then a neutralizer will stop the process. Three different strengths are available to target different hair types: mild, medium, and coarse. Estrada advises stopping by the salon to retouch the newly grown hair every six to eight weeks to ensure that hair is in good condition and steering clear of relaxers if your hair is already colored or bleached.

Reverse perms, according to Estrada, are another option and use liquid relaxing formulas instead of heavy creams. "Reverse perms relax your curl so it stays straight when you blow-dry your hair, but if you decide to let your hair dry naturally, you end up with a totally softened curl," she says. "This is great for people with soft wavy or soft curly hair who want to soften their curl, make it appear longer, and take out the frizz and can be redone every three to four months to maintain the look and texture of your hair." The big news in hair straightening these days is the Japanese straightening system, which is only available in salons. Chemicals are applied to the hair to relax it and then a flat iron is used to totally kill your curls so that you can wash hair, let it dry, and it remains completely straight for up to a year. Imagine how much more free time you'll have without having to blow-dry.

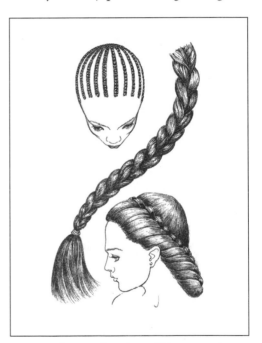

Braiding can be a beautiful, neat, and classic way to style longer hair.

The Braid Brigade

Centuries ago, people used to keep their hair under control by braiding it and keeping it close to the head in a decorative style. These days, new techniques and styles have made braiding popular again.

Think back to arts-and-crafts hour at summer camp. "Braiding is like macramé," says Paul Labrecque, of the Paul Labrecque Salon in New York. "But instead of using rope to make knots you are twisting hair together using two or more strands of hair to make interesting shapes on the head."

There are many types of braids: two-stranded braids, three-stranded braids, fishtails, French braids, inverted cornrows, the list goes on. To extend the length of your hair and give it a completely different look, fake hair can be added to your own hair and interlocked in a braid. Braids can be left loose on the head or can hug it tight to add style or create an interesting look. Before you leave the salon, make sure braids aren't too tight or they will feel uncomfortable and put a strain on your hair, causing breakage. But the looser the braids are, the more frequently you will need to have them done. Sometimes wet hair is braided and allowed to dry so that when the braid is removed, the hair has a crimped effect. This is a great way to style hair without using heat or chemicals and is less damaging. According to Labrecque, you can wash your hair and scalp once a week with braids in. If left in too long, braids may start to dreadlock and can damage hair. If your scalp starts to itch or flake while your braids are in, pour some SeaBreeze or witch hazel on a cotton ball and dab it on your scalp to take away the itch and dry, flaky skin.

We no longer have to settle for the type of hair we have—we can straighten it, curl it, color it, highlight it, or even braid it. But sometimes we are looking for a quick and temporary change that won't necessarily need to grow out. Like shopping for the latest trend, we want to try out a new color or style without having to commit to that look for a long period of time.

In Transition: How to Camouflage Your Growing Color

"The level of maintenance your hair requires depends a lot on the color of your natural hair and how dramatic the color is that you add to it," says Leslie Louise, hair colorist, Miwa Alex salon in New York City. "When I'm talking to clients about the color they want, maintenance is an essential topic. A good color job should last about six weeks, but it really depends on the individual and how fast her hair grows."

The bottom line: Those last couple of weeks before your next appointment can be brutal. Women have been known to try everything to camouflage their color, even coloring the hair at the roots with eye shadow or mascara in the same color family as their processed hair! Bad idea. These products were not made for your hair. Your best bet? Follow these tried-and-true maintenance tips:

- If you usually get your hair highlighted, have a single process done twice before you make an appointment for highlights again to lighten the base. "It's better for your hair," says Louise, "less costly, and easier to maintain the color."

- Ask your colorist about color shampoos and conditioners, which tend to deposit a little color into new growth to create the appearance of a little more color at the base. "This will help take you through a few more weeks," says Louise.

- Try highlighting shampoos and conditioners. They contain peroxide which, says Louise, can lighten your hair when you use a blow-dryer or go out in the sun. "They're fairly mild but they lift the color just a little."

Chapter 5

Styling Enhancements

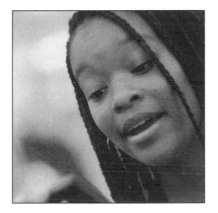

If you're not happy with the hair you were born with, don't let it get you down. There are plenty of styling options available for women who want a new look or who want to enhance the hair they have. Wigs, hairpieces, weaves, and extensions are all designed to transform your image or compensate for hair that needs a little extra augmentation. Here are the options and how they can give you the hair you love.

Wigging Out

Whether you wear them as a fashion statement or to cover up hair that is thinning or has fallen out, wigs can totally transform your look. On Broadway, women wear wigs to bring a character to life. In religion, women wear wigs to preserve their modesty and look good at the same time. In fashion, the runways are alive with women who really want to make a statement.

"Our clients are Broadway stars, actors, and medical referrals from hospitals like Sloan-Kettering," says Edward James Maloney, assistant manager and stylist at Barry Hendrickson's Bitz-n-Pieces in New York City. "When a customer comes in, a stylist consults with her in a private room to discuss the problems she is encountering with her hair and to try out different looks. Together they will decide what's right for her face and skin."

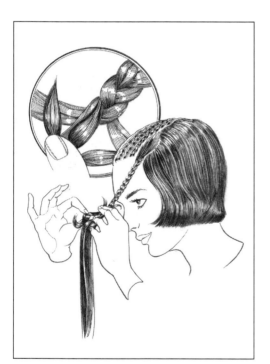

Weaving can extend the length of your hair and bolster its fullness.

Wigs are made from three types of materials: human hair, synthetic hair, and a blend of the two. According to Maloney, human hair is nicer to the touch and looks the most natural, but synthetic hair is easier to style. The combination gives you the best of both worlds, but you have to be happy with the texture of the wig and find the one that will work for you. Most women buy a wig that most closely resembles the texture of their natural hair.

The next thing that needs to be decided is the method of attachment, since there are several options to choose from. Wigs can be attached with toupee tape if there is no hair on the head, with little clips that snap and lock onto the hair whether there is a good amount of fully grown hair or still a sufficient amount of thinning hair, or with less secure bobby pins or clips, which are fastened to the wig liner. A head ped, or flat cap, holds the hair in place underneath the wig and keeps it flatter so that the wig sits on the head more snugly.

Next, the wig is fitted to the shape of the head and will be cut and styled to create each woman's own individual look. Most women opt for a style that is similar to one they are used to. "If a woman is getting a wig for medical reasons, she is going through enough already and has no time for an identity crisis. She wants to be able to recognize herself," says Maloney. As always, price is a factor. Human hair is the most expensive, almost double or triple that of synthetic hair.

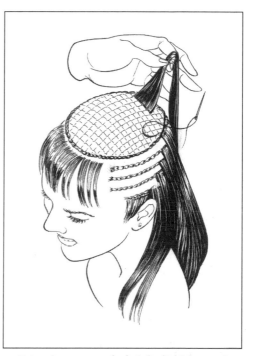

Extensions can make hair look thicker and more versatile in terms of styling options.

For financial reasons, most women end up buying a wig that's a human/synthetic blend. They return once every three weeks to have their wigs styled, and since they have to leave their wigs at the shop to be air-dried overnight—a process that is gentler on the material than blow-drying—they need to have a second wig or a suitable scarf or hat to wear in the meantime.

Being fit for a wig is only half the battle. "Female pattern baldness, or alopecia, and having cancer are major issues, and it's a big step to have to finally admit you need a piece," says Maloney. "But when you get to that point, you have to jump into the water. Wearing a wig is all about attitude. You have to present yourself like you're playing an actress but the character you're creating is yourself." At Bitz-n-Pieces, customers learn how to put their wigs on and walk and stand in their wigs as if they are an extension of themselves or their own hair.

MYTH: Hair bands, clips, barrettes, and other ornaments will break hair.

FACT: Using rubber bands to pull hair back can tear or rip hair. However, covered or fabric bands and most plastic clips and barrettes are harmless to hair when used properly. It's the pulling of hair that is most damaging, not the use of products like these.

Get a Piece

Another option for women who experience hair thinning in the frontal region is hairpieces. Though less common among women than men, some women find they make their hair look fuller and blend so well with real hair that often they look more natural than a wig. Women who want to cover a smaller area and don't want to be restricted by a full wig often wear them. Hairpieces are made out of natural human hair to match the color, texture, natural wave, or straightness and thickness of real hair. Like wigs, less expensive versions can be made of animal hair or artificial fibers. One of the most popular methods of hair replacement, hairpieces can be costly depending on the materials used. It's also important to know that attaching a hairpiece can affect hair loss on the head underneath it as a result of the method of attachment that is used. Bonding with strong glue is the most abrasive method, while clips are the least damaging. Adhesive-attached hairpieces can leave a sticky residue on the scalp that needs to be washed off and can also be loosened by perspiration or water. Snaps can be sewn into the hair but must be relocated as hair grows out.

If your hairpiece is permanently attached, it must be removed every six weeks by a hairstylist or technician so that it can be cleaned and your hair and scalp can be properly shampooed to remove the accumulation of flaked-off skin cells, oil, and shed hair that accumulates between the hairpiece and the scalp.

Dream Weavers

Weaving is a process that allows strands of hair to be woven together to extend the length or fullness, or to attach another piece of hair. It is one of the processes used to secure hairpieces. Your own hair is pulled through the opening in the hairpiece foundation and woven through it to secure the hairpiece to your head. The good news: This makes the hairpiece very secure through many points of attachment. The bad news: Weaves can cause traction alopecia, localized premature hair loss caused by the pulling of the hair in that area. Usually, through hair weaving, the hairpiece is tied to your natural hair with a tough, non-shrinkable thread and the two are woven together to form anchoring points for the piece. A trained hairdresser knows how to regularly remove the piece to have it washed and dried and is able to offer periodic tightening, which is required to keep the hair weave in place as hair continues to grow.

In addition to weaving in hairpieces, weaving can also be used to attach braids and extensions. According to Paul Labrecque, women who have cornrows often opt to attach braids or extensions over the rows to make hair look longer. The process of weaving involves sewing an additional weft of hair tightly to a braid or twist. It can take approximately two hours and will last a month before the braid grows away from the hair and has to be tightened.

Extend Yourself

Extensions can make your hair look thicker and can help you make a fashion statement at the same time. To get longer, very natural-looking hair, try extensions that match the color and texture of your hair. If you want a style-setting twist, choose from funky colors and synthetic textures, which give you a cutting-edge identity and make heads turn.

Extensions can be added to your own hair through weaving, sewing, bonding with glue or protein polymers. Anyone can wear them. They can get expensive when applied all over your head—just ask African-American women, who are known for using extensions to extend their cornrows or shorter braids. Women with thicker hair can get away with cheaper options. But if you have thinner hair, the extension hair will be more noticeable and the best quality hair should be used to keep it looking natural. Also, when adding extensions to fine hair, they should be sewn tightly into the braid so that little pieces that may stick out can't be seen. No matter what type of extensions you choose, Labrecque says it's all about maintenance. If you don't take care of your hair, it will be totally damaged and knotted and the only way to get the knots out will be to cut them off. To make sure your extensions are being properly attached and maintained, do your homework. Ask around to find a stylist who has a good reputation for putting them in. If a stylist has been written up positively in a magazine or if you have seen his/her work on a friend, there's a good chance the work he/she does on you will look great, too. Extensions can take up to six or seven hours if the stylist creates tiny cornrows first and then adds the extensions to them. Extensions alone can take about four hours; so make sure you really want them before you make the investment. If you do decide to go through with it, your hair will be hassle-free for some time. Extensions can be left in until the hair grows out as long as they are periodically maintained. Often they can get heavy and pull on the hair, so they need to be tightened or redone every three to four weeks.

Part Two

Common Hair Problems

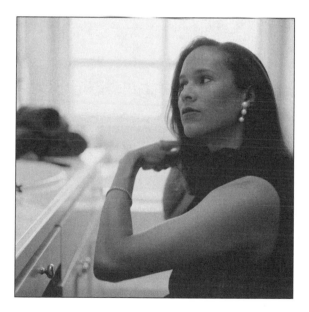

Chapter 6

Tackling the Environment, Hair Products, and Bad Habits

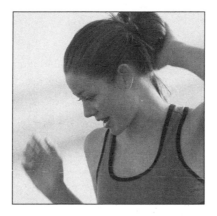

If we could keep the texture and color of the hair we were born with, we would be spared lots of hassles in later years. But the rigors of daily life—some a result of the abuse we inflict on our hair and others brought about by Mother Nature herself—can really take their toll. This chapter carefully examines what actually happens when our hair is exposed and how we can prevent damage in the future.

Environmental Enemies

A quick look at the vinyl fading away on the body of an old car is proof that environmental factors can cause a significant amount of damage. Sun, wind, pollution, chlorine, salt water, mold, and fungus can strip away hair's protective coating and leave it exposed to battle the elements. What's really happening? The sun may feel warm and soothing on your hair, but it actually breaks down the bonds that form the cuticle until the inner coil unfolds, then splits or breaks. If your hair is permed or colored, direct sunlight can act as an oxidant and fade the color in just a few hours. According to Pat Peterson at Aveda, wearing a hat and being prudent about keeping your hair covered can help limit the exposure and cause minimal damage. Styling products with antioxidants also help protect hair by sealing the cuticle. This fights off dryness and keeps hair moisturized. If you're in the sun, grease back your hair with sunblock or conditioner for extra protection. If you spend most of your time indoors, you are probably being exposed to harsh overhead lighting instead of full-spectrum lighting, which can have the same result as sunlight.

Abuse from wind is purely mechanical. Try driving down the highway in your new convertible sports car for an hour. It's fun to let your hair whip around uncontrollably and let your spirit soar, but you'll look like you've been through a windstorm

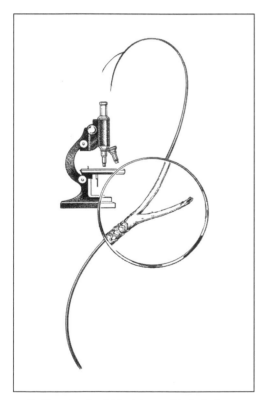

Split ends should be trimmed to help keep the hair healthy and in top condition.

by the end of your journey (think Renee Zellweger on her magical weekend getaway date with Hugh Grant in *Bridget Jones's Diary*). Even if you don't mind looking a bit disheveled, try getting all those knots out of your hair and you'll wish you had taken the train! What's really happening: Your cuticle is rough, so if you allow your hair to be roughened up, it will get tangled and break and cause split ends. The obvious solutions are tying hair back with a band or tucking it under a hat to keep it from getting mussed.

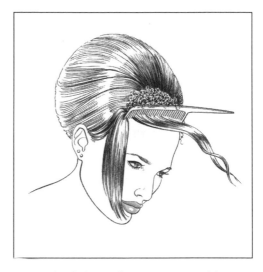

Teasing hair may be necessary to achieve certain looks, but it wreaks havoc on hair and should be done infrequently, if at all.

Another environmental problem is pollution. Just as moist skin attracts dirt and grime, the oil found on your hair attracts the same impurities. In fact, several studies have been done in regard to skin and hair in which scientists drew samples and found that natural oils were combined with hydrocarbons produced by car exhaust and other materials found in the air from petroleum sources. "Oil attracts grease, sulfites, and metals, which can coat hair and make it look dirty," says Peterson. "The best solution is to get a good shampoo and get rid of it." If you live in the desert, you know that hot air can dry out your hair. And if you live in a cold climate, you know that dry indoor heat from heaters that are turned on in the winter can also cause hair to lose moisture. In fact, we're all too familiar with bad hair days. Peterson says any atmosphere, whether it's dry or humid, will affect your hair, weakening the stabilizing bonds and temporarily restructuring your hair's style. Dry hair sucks moisture out of the air, leaving wispy, flyaway strands. If you straighten your hair, and the air is humid, water molecules push themselves into temporary bonds you

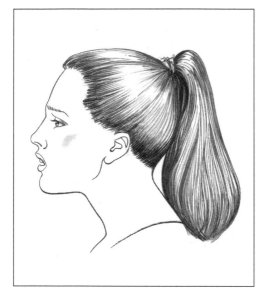

Plain rubber bands twisted tightly around the hair can damage and break delicate strands.

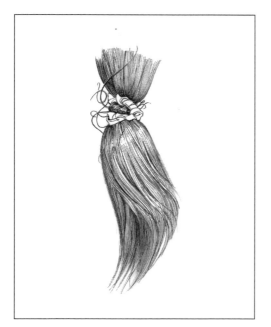

An untidy rubber band isn't just messy-looking, it's very unforgiving.

created by straightening and make hair revert back to the curvature nature gave it, leaving hair limp or frizzy. Salt water is another culprit when it comes to drying out your hair. The salt strips hair of its protective barrier, so it's important to rinse your hair immediately after a dunk in the ocean to preserve its moisture. Chlorine, made with bleach, which is a drying agent, is another one of hair's worst nightmares, causing the outside of the hair shaft to dry out and the center to be exposed. Chlorine also reacts with transition metals in water, changing the color of your hair. Black hair will typically turn green or orange; brown hair will take on an orange or red tint, and blond hair adopts a greenish hue. Swimmers should know this best: Spending large quantities of time in chlorinated water causes hair to become dry and brittle because the inside is exposed. The shafts weaken and often break. Urea and sodiumthiosulfate, two agents found in the popular swimmer's shampoo UltraSwim, bind with the chlorine and rinse it away. "If you don't wash your hair right away, the chlorine will sit on the hair and dry it out," explains Mike Davies, research and development manager for Chattem, the makers of UltraSwim shampoo and conditioner. "Any shampoo will do the trick if you use it right away but the longer you sit, the more you need a product that works hard to rinse away chlorine and restore hair's moisture."

Patronizing Products

Imagine what your hair goes through every day. In addition to basic washing and drying, it's subjected to brushes, combs, curling and straightening irons, barrettes, bands, clips, pins, creams, lotions, sprays, and oils. Here's a look at what to use and what to avoid if you want to keep your hair looking and

Accessory Test

Are your hair accessories hurting your hair? If you wear rubber bands for ponytails, slip one on your wrist before putting it in your hair. If it pulls your skin, it will pull your hair. To test a banana clip, place the clip on a couple of fingers. If it practically pinches off your circulation, it will damage your hair, too. Cotton is a great material to use on your hair, not rubber. The rule of thumb: If it doesn't feel good on bare skin, it's not good for your hair. Plastic isn't so bad, but if it's bound by a metal spring, make sure the spring isn't too tight. The more natural fiber a product is made of, the less tight it feels.

feeling its best. "You can spend as much time damaging your hair as you can being careful," says Carrie White, creative director and hair stylist at the Tova salon, Beverly Hills, California. "You can rip through three times quickly or comb through once slowly and carefully. The focus should be on how you are doing what you're doing." White says that combing isn't even necessary unless you wear your hair curly. As soon as you come out of the shower, comb through hair with a large rake comb so it doesn't dry in a knot or snarl. Then diffuse hair and pump it up with your hand to make it big and curly. One of most common ways to damage your hair is by over blow-drying it with a dryer that's too hot. If you choose a flat iron for straightening and smoothing hair, don't keep it pressed on the hair for five minutes. Instead, lift it through the hair to straighten it. The bottom line, adds White: "You can have the best tools in the world and be abusive if you're negligent in your activity with them." White advises using combs only when they are new and throwing them away after a good number of uses so that they don't break.

Irritating Accessories

Even accessories that are meant to make hair look glamorous can wreak havoc if they're not hair-worthy. According to Brad Johns, New York–based gold and silver jewelry designer, hairdresser, and colorist, it's important to make sure the pieces don't damage the hair. Bobby pins should have rubber tips. Check the closures to make sure they offer the right amount of tension. "If the back of a barrette is too tight, it will rip apart wet or dry hair, or squeeze and bend it until it's ready to break. Banana clips should be outlawed altogether. Not only are they tacky, but you can also ruin your hair with the metal springs. If a ponytail is too tight, hair is vulnerable. Tension rubber bands sit on the hair fibers and rip them out. Choose a terry cloth ponytail band instead." Johns creates geometric and sculptural pieces to contrast hair's soft waves, or amorphous pieces that blend in with the sculpture of the hair.

Sticky Solutions

Want to run your fingers through your significant other's locks? Beware. While some products can really make your hair look amazing, others can leave it looking and feeling sticky and stiff. "Great products alleviate all that and give you softness and shine," says White. "Lighter products have less weight and can change the texture and style of your hair." Read the ingredients; products with high alcohol levels can permeate the hair shaft and damage hair.

Again, understand your hair type before you apply. Straight hair often means static, so use products that coat and smooth the hair shaft; a lotion combed through towel-dried hair tames flyaways, moisturizing products combat the frizzies. Tightly curled hair can look dull; comb a moisturizing styling cream or paste through wet hair to calm the cuticle while defining the curl; straightening balm eliminates frizz at the hairline; silicone serums seal the cuticle to give curls dimension without weighing them down. For wavy hair, it's important to relax the hair shaft with smoothing spray and work through hair from roots to ends with a wide-tooth comb. Creams or non-sticky styling gels polish and add hold. For fine hair, massage medium-hold products into hair with your fingers to plump the hair shaft; use oil-free finishing products on the ends.

Overshampooing can leave buildup on your hair and can be hard on the hair shaft, so stick to the once-a-day or once every-other-day rule. Contrary to popular belief, it's not necessary to reshampoo in order to restyle. Instead, stand in the bathroom for a few minutes with the shower on to make your hair pliable enough to rework, then fine-tune with a round brush and a hairdryer. For curly hair, wet hair with warm water from a spray bottle, apply new product on hands and run them through your hair, and style as normal. Don't do this more than once or twice, or buildup will weigh hair down and you will need to start over and wash your hair completely.

Playing Games

"Twisting and chewing breaks hair and damages it from the roots up. Even cutting the ends won't help at that point," says New York City salon owner Yves Durif, of women who bite, twist, tease, and pull. Many of us play with our hair when we get nervous, says the stylist, which is a bad habit that needs to be broken.

"People who play with their hair all the time know that it's the top and front sections that are the most fragile," says Durif. "These are the

How to Keep Your Brush Clean

How often you clean your brush depends on how often you brush your hair and how much product you use. The general rule: Once every two to three weeks, mix a teaspoon of shampoo into a basin of warm water and dip brush bristles up to the cushion in the water. Swirl it around then shake off excess water and lay it on its back to dry.

areas that are affected most by the oxygen in the air and the sweat on your hands that is transferred to your hair when you push it back off your face." Sweat, explains Durif, can be abrasive to hair because of its alkalinity, weakening and attacking hair. Curly hair is drier by nature and more fragile than straight hair. It can really be damaged during a shampoo. Too much shampoo can be abrasive (once a day is more than plenty), and if the shampoo isn't rinsed out properly, the conditioner won't get its job done. Also, combing through hair with shampoo on it results in tangles. Homemade highlights, in the form of pure peroxide, leave the hair shaft exposed. Sometimes pulling your hair can be more than just a nervous twitch. Six to eight million people in the U.S. population, more women than men, have the repetitive urge to pull out their hair, causing noticeable bare spots, an excessive compulsive neurobiological disorder called trichotillomania. Christina Pearson, the executive director of the trichotillomania Learning Center in Santa Cruz, California, a national nonprofit education resource center, says there is no explanation for why people do it. Pulling is triggered by being too tired or overstressed and, says Pearson, the majority of women pull from the scalp, then eyelashes, brows, pubic hair, and elsewhere on the body. About 50 percent of the calls to the center are concerns about young children who are pulling their hair, and a third of all women and men who buy wigs have the disorder.

"The best treatment approach is to educate people about what it is," says Pearson, who grew up with the disorder since her teens, "and to develop a behavioral approach to control it." Through her program, Pearson tries to help people retrain their nervous systems through behavioral therapy, either alone or combined with antidepressant drugs. Other treatments include hypnosis, dietary restrictions, support groups, traditional therapy, and acupuncture. She says that any way of de-stressing the nervous system is helpful. "Dietary changes, such as reducing your sugar and caffeine intake, which can agitate the nervous system, can help." Through the Trichotillomania Learning Center, Pearson and her staff work to educate people about the disorder through conferences and symposiums, provide referrals for treatment, and offer help through a scientific advisory board that consists of leading clinicians and researchers who help the organization stay on the cutting edge of treatment.

Tools of the Trade

You can have the most beautiful hair in the world, but if you don't treat it right, it won't stay that way for long. Our experts teach you how to brush, comb, curl, straighten, iron, and set your hair while keeping it healthy.

Brush Biz

"Many people don't realize there is such a thing as the right hairbrush," says Elizabeth Manoughian, president, Jean-Pierre Creations, who advises purchasing one brush to dry hair and another to style. "Good quality, design, and suitability to hair length, texture, and styling needs are the most important qualities when it comes to choosing a brush." Mason Pearson brushes have been put to the scalp since 1895, specifically for grooming purposes, according to Robert Sansone, the company's national sales director. "The design is simple," says Sansone, "all pneumatic suction brushes are slightly domed with bristles that sit on a cushion of air to conform to the cushion of your head while brushing. They're made of 100 percent natural rubber and the handles are composed of molded acrylic resin." According to Sansone, boar bristle is the material that's closest to human hair in structure and composition so it won't cause damage. It's not overly stiff and has a smooth surface and cuticle—perfect for distributing sebum from the sebaceous gland. "There is no other mechanical process that can be performed across the hair shaft to distribute oil, which nature gives us for supple, elastic, shiny, and healthy hair while exfoliating the scalp and stimulating the hair follicle."

MYTH: Brushing 100 strokes a night is great for hair growth, shine, and health.

FACT: Vigorous nightly brushing can do more harm than good to hair's health. It can also stimulate oil glands that can lead to oily, flat hair.

There are four brush sizes to choose from and each size has a pure boar-bristled head or bristles with nylon spikes. Use the pure bristled brush for short hair and the nylon-spiked bristle brush for textured or thick hair.

A good brush should be gentle yet stimulating and easily glide through the hair. From boar to synthetic, barrel to paddle, Elizabeth Manoughian offers these guidelines.

- Make sure the handle is made of durable, high-grade wood or plastic and fits comfortably in your hand. A well-designed brush is never clunky or awkward.

- Opt for the highest-grade bristles you can get. Inexpensive boar bristle brushes often use a cheaper quality cut of boar bristle, which is too supple for effective brushing, while high-quality synthetic brushes are smooth and cleanly cut to prevent them from scratching the scalp or yanking out hair.

- For thick or curly hair, try a brush made of a mixture of boar and nylon bristles to penetrate highly textured hair.

- For everyday brushing, a large-surface paddle brush is the best option. Blow-dry with a round brush (the wider the barrel, the larger the curl).

- Maximum bristle density and high row count provide a more solid, even surface, which creates optimum tension for faster blow-drying and easier smoothing.

- Straightening brushes clamp hair tight like a straightening iron, so it's easier to pull curl out as you blow-dry.

- Boar bristles smooth frizz on fine to normal hair, and they make hair look shiny and are gentle to the scalp.

- Vent brushes allow warm air to pass through them directly to the root and speed up drying time since the metal conducts heat to facilitate drying.

- Try a tiny, small-barreled round brush for styling and curling shorter hair.

- Try a nylon-boar combination brush for short, thick to normal hair. It offers better grab for styling, adds shine, and reduces frizz.

- Use a nylon brush to pull tangled strands through coarse, thick hair.

- Go for a metal brush to bring shine back to highlighted hair. It conducts heat from the hair and seals the cuticle.

The Comb Connection

"Generally speaking, there are two kinds of widely used combs," says Bertrand Thiery, general manager for J. F. Lazartigue. "Large-tooth combs with eight to ten teeth have no other role than to detangle hair and prepare it for blow-drying. Short-tooth combs are very narrow with tiny, one-inch tall teeth and are mostly used by men to comb their hair in the right direction. The ends of the teeth are square so they don't touch and irritate the scalp. Longer widths with softer, round-edged teeth touch and massage the scalp. "These days," says Thiery, "if a woman owns a comb, it's used for teasing hair to get volume. This technique was used a lot in the 1950s, but women who still seek volume will resort to it. A brush is softer and less damaging to the hair." The biggest mistake women make when combing their hair, according to Thiery, is to use a narrow-tooth comb to detangle hair when wet. "If hair is ready to break, a brush will cause less damage." Women with afros or kinky hair often use a pick or a wide-tooth comb to style hair without breaking the curl, says Thiery. A brush won't work because the teeth aren't long enough and won't get down to the roots. Since most combs directly touch the scalp, use 60 percent alcohol to kill fungus and disinfect your comb at least once a month.

The Heat of the Matter

Some of the best options for styling your hair involve heat—a great tool for making your hair look its best in the short term, a culprit in causing all kinds of damage in years to come. No matter which styling tool you decide to use, hold it a good distance away from hair or keep the heat directly on hair for only a few seconds at a time. And if you're not going anywhere special on a particular day, don't add unnecessary heat to your hair. Give it a break and let it air-dry. That said, check out these styling options designed to help you get the looks you love:

Curling irons are the best way to get any kind of curl. Use a 1-inch iron with a shortened clamp for spiral curls, a medium-barrel iron for loose waves, or a large-barrel iron for more volume. First, let hair air-dry. Insert the end of a section into the clamp then wind the rest of the section of hair into a spiral up the length of the barrel. Hold for three to four seconds, unwrap, and repeat. Vary the tension and direction of the curl for a less "done" look.

Waving irons give hair softer "s"-shaped waves. Blow-dry hair and separate into 2-inch sections. Start at the crown of your head, clamp iron at the root of one section, hold for three to five seconds, release, and move down the hair shaft, continuing around the head.

Straightening irons are every wavy-haired woman's dream come true. For long, curly hair, choose an iron that offers 135–170 watts of heat and has long, wide panels, which make it easier to straighten long hair quickly. For fine, frizzy hair, 40-watt versions are sufficient to straighten hair without flattening it or causing frizz or damage. Smaller versions of the straightening iron are easier to maneuver on short hair and are ideal for bangs, short layers around the hairline, and for styling ends.

Winter Woes

When cold weather hits, you probably notice that your hair starts to behave differently. It tends to dry out and becomes hard to manage. Luckily, there are lots of little things that you can do to protect it. Here are a few expert tips for treating dry winter hair:

- Don't wash your hair too often during the winter months. Use a dry shampoo once or twice a week to give it a break.

- Moisturize your hair with a leave-in conditioner and conditioning heat-activated hairspray.

- Don't go outside with your hair wet or you risk freezing your hair, which may result in breakage.

- For extra protection from the elements, wear a hat or wrap a scarf around your head.

- Pump a drop of body lotion onto your hands and rub them together, then run them through your hair to smooth over flyaway strands and help eliminate static cling.

How to Un-Roll

Gripping Velcro rollers can take your hair out with them as you unroll. If you get one stuck in your hair, advises Yves Durif, put some conditioner on the hair and try to comb it out with a big, thick comb, pulling a few strands at a time.

"Ninety-six percent of American homes have a blow-dryer, but it's important to blow-dry your hair as little as possible to help retain moisture and not dry it out," says New York hairstylist David Kinigston, creative consultant for Jean Pierre Creations.

First, choose your weapon. Consider power wattage, size, compactness, ergonomic features, and other characteristics that pertain specifically to the type and texture of your hair. Circular airflow diffusers give curly hair volume and lift without frizz, while a cool-shot button helps smooth hair. Multiple heat and speed settings help minimize damage, and the quick-dry version with twin barrels maximizes airflow. Ionic stylers reduce the size of water droplets and allow more moisture to be absorbed into the cuticle to eliminate flyaways and reduce static when straightening. Built-in nozzles have 20 percent more concentrated air than other hair-dryers, and special fan designs make some dryers up to 75 percent quieter to suit early risers who don't want to wake the rest of the household. An 1875-watt dryer will last a good amount of time, depending on the amount of usage, and is great for thick hair; a 1500-watt dryer is fine for thinner hair; while a 1200-watt dryer isn't as powerful and won't last as long. Compact dryers with foldable handles are great to slip into a suitcase, but most hotels now have them in their rooms, so ask in advance.

Paulette Heller, director of marketing for hair-dryers at Conair, advises not to scrimp on cost or you will be buying a unit made of thinner plastic. Since it's the housing that protects your hair from the heat, a thinner model will grow hotter faster. Additionally she offers her do's and don'ts on hair-dryer care and usage.

- DO look for alternate setting options like high and low, so that you can control how hot the dryer will become.

- DO clean the lint buildup in back once a month so that the dryer doesn't overheat.

- DON'T stick any tools inside the filter to remove debris.

- DO roll up the cord or buy a unit with a retractable one to preserve the life of the cord.

- DON'T roll cord around the dryer, especially when it's still hot.

- DO keep your hair-dryer in a basket, on a shelf, or in a drawer. If your dryer has a hook attachment, you can hang it in your bathroom.

- DON'T store your hair-dryer near water.

To prep hair for a blow-dry, Eufora International artist Haim Knister advises squeezing your wet hair with a towel to dry, and combing hair through with a comb or brush from the bottom up. Then, vigorously dry hair with a blow-dryer, using your hands to lift hair up from underneath to get the moisture out. Turn off the dryer when hair is about 75 percent dry, apply volumizer or holding gel, turn the dryer to a lower setting, and you're ready to style.

The way to blow-dry hair is about as individualistic as the way you sign your name. According to Kinigston, here are the basics: Place your brush under a section of hair at the roots so the bristles are at the scalp. Hold the dryer at the roots for a few seconds, one to six inches away from your head so that it's not too close to the scalp and not directly on your hair, then rotate the brush slightly away from your head as you lift hair up and away from the roots, stroking down to the ends. Keep the dryer pointed down the hair shaft, following the motion of the brush. To straighten hair, pull it taut while drying and bring the brush straight through to the ends. "A round or flat brush is ideal for controlling the direction and texture of your hair," adds Knister, who recommends allowing each section of hair to cool on the brush before moving to the next section. "Don't damage hair by continuously re-blowdrying sections." Finish with spray gel or wax for hold and definition.

Get Set

Lucky for you, you don't have to sit under a heat-infused shower cap attached to a machine with your hair rolled up in curlers all around your head like your grandmother used to. These days, getting a fresh new wave or adding body to your coif is as easy as a few strategically placed rollers and a matter of a few minutes at best. In fact, there are hundreds of brands of rollers on the market, so you may spend even more time deciding on which rollers to choose rather than actually setting your hair. Hot rollers give your hair instant, more definitive curls that last throughout the day. If you have more time, try Velcro rollers, which are less expensive and more convenient to use since you don't have to wait for them to get hot. The curl takes about ten minutes to set. Technologically advanced rollers are being constructed every day. A new brush and roller combination offers home stylists an all-in-one solution. There's a large round brush with six interchangeable barrels of different sizes that you can slide off and leave in your hair as you blow-dry. For best results, style hair right after drying when it's still warm, rolling 1- to 2-inch sections at a time away from your face, from front to back all over your head. Spritz with hairspray and allow to set for 15 minutes.

Chapter 7

How Medical Conditions Affect Hair and What You Can Do About Them

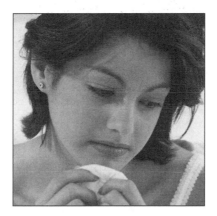

Sometimes having a bad hair day isn't simply a matter of an unruly wave or a little frizz. Occasionally, hair trouble can be a result of something else that's going on in your body. Medical conditions like metabolic dysfunction or illness can lead to thinning hair or hair loss or have some other, more subtle effect. Anemia, thyroid dysfunction, hormonal disturbances, and nutritional inadequacies affect hair the most, but unless other symptoms can be identified, it is difficult to recognize that hair problems are due to illness. The effects of fever, accidents, surgery, or pregnancy are other overlooked reasons for hair trouble. Too often physicians chalk up the hair loss problem to genetics when it could be a result of illness or medication. So before you seek revenge on your hairstylist, you might want to give your doctor a call.

Thanks, Mom! It's All in Your Genes

So when is hair loss a genetic issue? "If a woman comes to see me, the first thing I ask is whether or not anyone in her family has been affected by hair thinning or loss," says Dr. Shelly Friedman, president of the American Board of Hair Restoration Surgery, who claims his grandmother suffered from the problem but no one could ever tell since she always wore her hair up. "Your hair gets its longevity from one side of your family and its texture and color from another, so you can have curly hair that's destined to live forever or straight hair that's destined to die by thirty-five. If the woman tells me no other female members of her family have hair loss, then I look at the possible medical reasons."

Rx for Your Tresses: Medical Conditions and Your Hair

As if it isn't horrifying enough to be diagnosed with a medical condition, imagine being diagnosed with a problem that cites hair loss as a side effect. Though modern science is rapidly plugging away to find a solution, sometimes the hair issue can't even be treated, because the treatment could interfere with the medications you are taking for the initial problem.

Philip Kingsley says, below-normal hemoglobin levels and below-average levels of iron storage can make your hair thin. A well-balanced diet, including vitamins and supplements, can help reverse the effect.

Kingsley, who also studied PCOS (polycystic ovarian syndrome), noticed an incidence of women's hair loss with the disorder. In a study of women in London, 68 percent of women with thin hair had PCOS. Stress, which seems to be the root of all of our problems these days, is actually one of the biggest reasons for hair loss. Experts say that stress produces adrenaline, which can lead to the production of cholesterol and testosterone. If your hair follicles are sensitive to testosterone, hair thinning can occur.

Lupus, an autoimmune disease, develops antibodies to its own cells and can, therefore, form antibodies to cells in the hair follicle.

Most common in middle-aged women, neurodermatitis is recognized by hard, patchy scaling above the nape of the neck at the base of the scalp. It itches drastically and scratching only makes it worse. Often confused with dandruff, neurodermatitis can go untreated. Kingsley suggests trying antidandruff shampoo or sulfur and salicylic acid cream or seeing a dermatologist for more advanced care.

Pityriasis amientacea is a thick scaling common in women in their forties and fifties and consists of adherent flakes climbing up the hair shaft. While often misdiagnosed, if treated correctly, it can be cured, but when neglected, it can cause hair loss.

Contact dermatitis is a recurrent scaly condition caused by an allergy to a certain product, like hair color. Since it usually flares up after the product has been applied, it is often easy to recognize.

Some other scalp conditions, according to Kingsley, may also be present but are extremely rare. Various folliculitis is an inflammation of the hair follicles caused by infection or the long-term use of a greasy product on the scalp. Rosacea can show up on the scalp in red blotches. And lichen simplex is a thickening of the skin on the scalp, caused by constant rubbing of the skin when it's itchy and flaky. In all cases, Kingsley advises immediate treatment by a professional.

According to Jeffrey Epstein, M.D., D.A.C.S., a doctor in private practice in Miami, Florida, diet binges are another culprit. Excessive dieting or eating disorders can cause a nutritional deficiency, which may limit the transport of nutrients to the scalp and cause hair follicles to die and fall out.

Of all the medical conditions and treatments that alter the state of the body and may cause hair loss, the most well known is chemotherapy, which is a common treatment for most types of cancer. It causes the most drastic of hair conditions—from balding in certain areas to complete hair loss.

"When cancer is present, the cancerous cells grow at a higher rate and replicate too quickly," explains Dr. Robert Guida, director of facial and plastic surgery at New York Weill Cornell Medical Center. "Chemotherapy causes cell destruction by blocking the cells and keeping them from regenerating. Cancer cells pick up chemotherapy agents quicker than normal cells but healthy cells are also affected. In addition, the toxins from the chemotherapy are damaging to the hair follicles." Scientists are now studying genes that they hope will be used one day to make chemotherapy agents specific to particular cancer cells to prohibit them from affecting different areas of the body.

Hormonal Havoc: Getting Your Hair Through Pregnancy, Nursing, and Menopause

Any woman who has encountered hormonal changes, whether in the form of puberty, pregnancy, or menopause, knows that hormones drastically affect us physically and emotionally. Hair loss is no exception. In pregnancy, mild degrees of hirsutism, male patterns of hair growth, can be found, making the proportion of hair in the growing phase during pregnancy lighter than that in the resting phase. "Certain hormones make hair follicles fall out as a group in a particular area, while normal follicles tend to fall out in separate intervals," explains Albert George Thomas, clinical associate professor of OB/GYN and director of family-planning services at Mount Sinai School of Medicine in New York City. "In the process, neighboring hair will cover empty spaces where hair has been lost. The process is reversed when hair grows and it's time for the alternate hair to fall out." Thomas, who is careful not to minimize the effects on the occasional patient who has severe hair loss, adds that while certain drugs might help retard the loss of hair on the scalp, gynecologists don't recommend using any medications during pregnancy even if it seems like the benefits will far outweigh any risks.

Hair loss is also seen during the postpartum period for about three to four months following delivery. "In pregnancy, there are high levels of estrogen and progesterone, which are responsible for hair loss," says Thomas. "In the postpartum phase, when breast-feeding is on demand around the clock, estrogen levels are lowered and eventually return to normal and hair grows back." Normal hair growth will occur six to fifteen months postpartum and it's usually not as thick as it was before pregnancy. This shedding process represents the reactivation of the hair follicle followed by new growth. "Some women are put on birth control pills to help stabilize postpartum hormonal balance and stimulate hair regrowth," says Sharon Weiner, M.D., a Los Angeles–based OB/GYN. "The nursing period is still a time of fluctuation."

MYTH: Women experience hair thinning the same way men do.

FACT: Unlike men, who get bald spots, women experience diffused thinning, particularly in the crown and temporal areas of the scalp.

Weiner says it's difficult to know how each woman reacts to oral contraception. "Some say their hair feels better, and gets thicker and stronger, while others say they feel their hair is thinning," she says. "It's a matter of individualizing the pill and finding the rate of estrogen and progesterone that's right for each woman." Menopause and perimenopause bring about other issues. In menopause, the amount of estrogen decreases and the level of androgens increases. "This concentric recruitment makes all of the hair follicles fall out as a group," says Thomas.

"Postmenopause, there is a fine balance between estrogen and testosterone, which comes with an elevated risk of heart disease, osteoporosis, and hair loss," says Dr. Epstein. "There is often a greater percentage of testosterone compared to estrogen, which may not be an actual elevation in testosterone but merely a depression or decrease in estrogen levels." "Women face many hair problems as they go through menopause and we are undertaking extensive research right now to learn more about it," says Dr. Weiner, who says she is hearing complaints of hair loss from women even under the age of forty. She is currently investigating the combination of hormones and genetics and their effects on hair loss to advise patients better on which combination of hormones to take.

MYTH: Stress causes permanent hair loss.

FACT: Although it's true that stress can be a factor in the temporary thinning of hair, it has no lasting effect on the condition of the hair. Once stress is treated, thinning no longer occurs as a symptom of that condition.

The Great Depression

Hair loss can be a devastating thing, both physically and emotionally. So it's understandable why many women who experience it often seek counseling to soothe their state of mind. Unfortunately, there aren't many proven treatments available. According to a panel of mental health experts reporting in the February 1997 *Journal of the American Medical Association,* depression has been undertreated in the United States, either because doctors don't have the necessary training to effectively treat it or because they may not view the condition seriously enough. Some studies have shown that only one in ten Americans with depression receive adequate treatment. When left untreated, depression can interfere with personal relationships and job performance and can increase your risk for other illnesses, according to a panel organized by the National Depressive and Manic Depressive Association. It's the fourth-leading public health problem in the world, yet only one in every three people suffering from depression ever seeks help.

"One of most traumatic situations for a woman to deal with is when she starts losing her hair," says Aleta St. James, a New York City–based emotional healer, who councils women on what they can do about it. "As a woman, this is a very difficult challenge, but there are ways around it." On a practical level, St. James suggests that women get a wig to wear until their hair starts to grow in again to make them feel pretty and attractive. In addition, she recommends concentrated efforts that will emotionally and spiritually help them release feelings that if they aren't pretty, they are unlovable. "I try to help women deal with their self-consciousness, the feeling that everyone is looking at them because there's something wrong with them," says St. James. "I try to teach them how to release that idea and understand that most people have empathy." Her advice: When you start to feel someone is looking at you as if they think there's something wrong with you, take a deep breath and release that feeling; then declare to yourself that the spirit in you honors the spirit in them. This will help make you feel connected to people rather than feeling separated from them and will give you a sense of calmness. "Reframe your relationship with these people," she adds. "Instead of seeing them as enemies or people who criticize you and make you feel small, see them as being connected to you in spirit." To test-drive St. James's mood-lifting techniques, try this visualization exercise: Close your eyes and visualize a gold-colored light coming into the top of your head. Concentrate on your negative feeling strongly and breathe that gold light into the part of your body where the feeling is stuck. Hold for a count of three and release. If you can visualize the gold light and pair it with the breath in your chest, heart, or throat area, you have targeted the grief. As you release your breath and the color, release your negative emotion. On the next inhale, think of something that gives you a strong feeling of love and draw that feeling into your body. Continue until the negative feeling has completely disappeared. Think about parts of yourself that you feel are attractive and embellish on those to obtain a true positive light.

St. James acknowledges that you may not be the only one who needs help in this department. "If someone is being critical of you, instead of feeling diminished and closed down, send them love," she continues. "Realize that most of these people would probably be terrified if this happened to them. Think of a pink sun right in your heart and send it to the person. This will stop you from feeling bad and from trying to defend yourself and make you realize that you can make a difference in their lives."

This Is Your Hair—On Drugs

The next time you pop an aspirin, take a good look in the mirror first. Even this common medication can cause scalp flaking, itching, and inflammation. If you are prone to asthma, hay fever, or eczema, you may even be more exposed to these effects. In fact, many routinely prescribed prescription and nonprescription drugs can cause temporary hair loss, aggravate female pattern baldness, trigger its onset, and cause permanent hair loss. Ask your physician if you can substitute one of these medications for a drug that doesn't have hair-loss side effects or use a natural treatment instead.

Acne drugs like Accutane, a derivative of vitamin A, may cause extensive drying of the scalp and other body surfaces, resulting in hair loss. The average prescribed dosage is often taken over the course of sixteen weeks, but a substantial amount of hair falls out toward the final weeks and usually grows back afterward.

Antibiotics can cause redness, tenderness, and flaking of the scalp if used over a long period of time. Anticoagulants like panwarfin, sofarin, coumadin, and heparin injections block clotting factors, so some believe they increase circulation to bring nutrients to the scalp.

Birth control pills contain hormones like estrogen, which can improve the appearance of your hair. Stop taking birth control pills, and there's a chance you could experience hair loss. But don't despair; it will only last about six months. Hormone-containing drugs and drugs prescribed for hormone-related reproductive conditions can potentially cause hair loss. Hormone replacement therapy (HRT) for postmenopausal women contains estrogen and/or progesterone, which can be metabolized into androgenic compounds, such as testosterone; anabolic steroids and prednisone can have similar effects.

Cholesterol-lowering drugs and convulsion/epilepsy anticonvulsants can cause hair loss. Antidepression medications, including Prozac, Zoloft, and Paxil, amphetamines used for dieting, and antifungals also trigger hair loss. Beta-blocker drugs, used to treat glaucoma and high blood pressure, can make hair fall out. Anti-inflammatory drugs, including those prescribed for localized pain, swelling, and injury, can help reduce scalp inflammation and help hair grow. Levadopa, administered for Parkinson's disease, can cause hair loss, too.

When it comes to thyroid imbalances, common treatment drugs such as Eltroxin Â (synthroid) and Tertroxin Ä (euthroid) need to be monitored carefully because an overdose or underdose can cause hair loss. Sedatives, tranquilizers, and barbiturates, taken over a long period of time, can cause redness or flaking of the scalp as well as thinning hair. Some also cause the scalp to be extra sensitive to sunlight. Many drugs used to treat stomach difficulties and ulcers can also affect hair loss.

Vitamins, often only thought of as beneficial, can also have some negative effects when it comes to your hair. Excessive doses of vitamin A (anything over 2,500 i.u. a day to 5,000 i.u. maximum) can make hair fall out. In addition, large doses of vitamin C can result in redness, flakiness, or itchiness of the scalp and skin, and vitamin E can prevent adequate iron absorption, leading to hair loss.

Once you realize that your hair is thinning or falling out, it's important to consider your treatment options, which include hair regrowth products, physical hair additions, and surgery.

Chapter 8

Scalp Problems and What You Can Do About Them

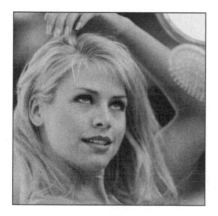

We've already determined that in order to have healthy hair, we need to maintain a healthy scalp. For this reason, it's important to understand the conditions that affect our scalp, mainly dandruff, psoriasis, and dry scalp, and to learn how we get them, how we can avoid them, and how we can clear up the mess if and when it occurs.

The Dirt on Dandruff

More than half of the U.S. population is affected by dandruff, a condition of the scalp in which a fungus called malassezia feeds on the skin's natural oils. For some women, overproduction of the fungus can cause scalp irritation, redness, and flaking, which can accelerate the body's normal shedding of dead skin cells and production of new ones. While the process usually takes 28 days, it can take as little as 7 to 10 days when dandruff is present. This revved-up rate produces scales that flake individually, so if you notice large white or gray flakes, itchiness, and either dryness in a specific area or excessive oiliness all over the scalp, there's a good chance you have dandruff.

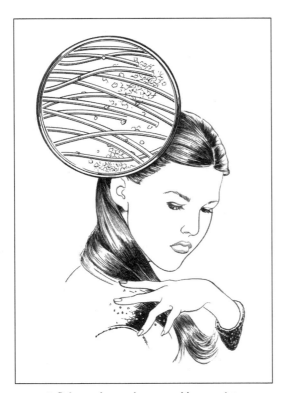

A flaky scalp can be caused by a variety of things, from overuse of hair products to hormonal changes to stress.

"Our skin cells shed all the time," explains Hilary Baldwin, associate professor of dermatology at the State University of New York at Downstate Medical Center. "In dandruff, cells are immature so they stick together and form greasy, visible patches of skin that can flake off and may be visible on your shoulders. With severe dandruff, your scalp may itch so much that the flakes can be scratched off at the most inopportune moments." Dandruff may get better or worse during any hormonal fluctuation, according to Baldwin, from puberty when women begin to produce more oils to pregnancy when hormonal levels are completely out of whack, to menopause when your scalp starts to dry out. "Stress can have a lot to do with dandruff and can make it less tolerable," she says.

You can have dandruff and an oily scalp, but more women find it associated with a dry one. A dry scalp is evident by smaller, more powdery flakes and a tight, itchy-feeling scalp and often becomes worse during the winter when the air is drier and the rest of your skin needs a little extra moisturizing, too. To avoid dry scalp, use a conditioning shampoo, refrain from shampooing every day, avoid heat from blow-drying, use a humidifier to combat indoor heat, and wear a hat to protect your head outside. Maintaining a healthy scalp will do more than keep you from having to deal with dandruff and dry scalp. "Other scalp problems include scalp

> ### Flaky Facts
>
> Turn your head upside down and brush or vigorously rub your scalp with your fingertips over a dark towel. If you see tiny, dry powdery flakes you have dry scalp. Use a clarifying shampoo with cider vinegar to remove buildup from products, and then try an oil treatment or scalp cream to moisturize. If the flakes are larger or look moist and greasy, you have dandruff. If the flakes are larger and look moist or greasy and your scalp is irritated, you may have seborrhea.

cysts, which have to be surgically removed if they become large enough, and scalp folliculitis, which is acne on the scalp," says Amy Beth Lewis, assistant clinical professor of dermatology at Downstate Medical Center and a New York–based dermatologist. "If you scratch often or start picking at the bumps, your scalp may bleed, and infections and other problems may occur." She says oral antibiotics offer a possible solution to curing the problem as well.

If you've been coloring, perming, relaxing, or straightening your hair, your scalp can become oily, flaky, and inflamed, which may mean you have a severe form of dandruff called seborrhea or seborrheic dermatitis, which can develop when the sebaceous glands are overactive as a result of emotional tension or poor diet. It can also turn up as a byproduct of an allergy, hormonal imbalance, or infection. Some studies show that dandruff is often related to poor metabolism of refined carbohydrates and a deficiency of B vitamins. Improving your diet and taking antioxidants may help the cause. If you treat it with a strong dandruff shampoo, it may only make it worse.

How to Deal with Dandruff

Unfortunately, you can be genetically predisposed to both seborreic dermatitis and psoriasis, and they can both be aggravated by stress, which causes additional scaling and flaking. A loss of moisture caused by certain styling habits such as blow-drying can also dry out your scalp. Here's how to smooth things over.

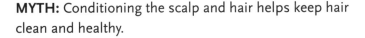

MYTH: Conditioning the scalp and hair helps keep hair clean and healthy.

FACT: Using conditioners on the scalp can actually clog pores. Conditioners should only be applied to hair, never to the scalp.

Not many women know that gentle shampoos that contain tea tree oil, rosemary, or sage can control damage without drying out your scalp or hair. Alternate with a dandruff shampoo or revise your daily hair care regimen to incorporate a shampoo with an antifungal ingredient that can get rid of flakes and keep new ones from forming. Some shampoos contain pyrithione zinc (ZPT) to help control and prevent dandruff. Others include selenium sulfide and ketoconazole, which reduce the amount of fungus on the scalp and help keep flakes from recurring. While approved by the FDA to fight dandruff, these ingredients may not be the best choices for great-looking hair and can leave your locks looking dried out, which will ultimately happen as you age. As you get older, the amount of sebum produced by the sebaceous glands diminishes, leaving your hair dry. To help retard this process, add two tablespoons of vegetable oil plus vitamin E and cod liver oil supplements to the daily diet, brush hair nightly, indulge in occasional pre-shampoo oil treatments, and refrain from shampooing more often than twice a week or try one of the following dandruff-controlling shampoos.

Pick Your Potion

If you'd rather have a root canal than be caught with a dandruff shampoo in your shower, you need to change your attitude. Some of the most effective dandruff shampoos can clear up your problem pronto, so they're worth the investment. Here's a look at the most well-known brands on the market. Products that contain pyrithione zinc as an active ingredient, like Head and Shoulders, are designed to kill the fungus that causes dandruff and help decrease irritation that's present with dandruff. "Women are afraid to strip color or perms from their hair or dry it out," says Baldwin. "Pyrithione zinc doesn't do that. And it's not a temporary solution. You can make it part of your hair- cleansing routine for life, especially now that there are different formulations for men, African-American hair, conditioners, and two-in-one versions to travel with or take to the gym." To make the product work better, Baldwin suggests getting out of the shower immediately after washing your hair, so you don't spend an excessive amount of time under the showerhead and wash the active ingredients down the drain. Head and Shoulders Intensive Treatment and Selsun Blue also contain selenium sulfide to help decrease the irritation that's present with dan-

Scalp Massage

As we've already determined, a healthy scalp is the basis for healthy hair. It's important to massage your scalp on a regular basis, starting at the nape of your neck and massaging upward with your spread fingertips moving in a slow circular motion. Follow by putting your fingers close together with one hand on each side of the top of your head, and zigzag back and forth from forehead to crown.

druff. A second over-the-counter option is a product with salicylic acid, which eats away at the thick, greasy scales so that flakes are less visible on your clothing after you shampoo. Ketoconazole is another ingredient that's reportedly effective in targeting the fungal overgrowth that causes dandruff. According to McNeil Consumer Healthcare in Pennsylvania, the company behind Nizoral A-D, which utilizes ketoconazole as a main ingredient, one in three Americans suffers from this embarrassing condition. Ketoconazole adheres to the scalp's natural proteins to provide protection and relief from dandruff for days in between washing. This is ideal for women who may skip a day or so between washing their hair. The formula also provides comfort and moisture to hair, making it shiny and manageable.

If over-the-counter brands don't get the job done, a doctor might prescribe a medicated shampoo that will. Capex shampoo, a topical corticosteroid with FDA approval for the treatment of severe dandruff, contains a low-potency topical steroid called fluocinolone acetonide to reduce inflammation and itching. "There are other topical steroids on the market in solution, foam, or lotion bases," says Mary Madden, senior product manager for Galderma, "but they often contain alcohol and have to be spot-treated and massaged into the part with your fingers. A shampoo formulation is the easiest way to uniformly distribute the product, get it to do what it needs to do, and conveniently rinse out." Capex shampoo cleanses scales, sebum, oil, and dirt from the hair and scalp while hydrating it so that solution can penetrate more effectively, and its anti-inflammatory properties cause a decrease in scaling, flaking, and itching.

Tar is another common antidandruff ingredient formulated to decrease the rapid turnover of skin cells. Neutrogena T-Gel is one such formula designed to reduce scaling without any strong anti-inflammatory activity and few surfactants to keep lathering to a minimum. It's ideal for women with scalp diseases who don't want to introduce another disorder. A word of caution: Some tar-based shampoos can smell bad and may dry out your hair.

Moisturizing oils and steroid drops are another combination treatment.

According to Lewis, oils applied to the scalp and left on overnight with a shower cap can cut through scaly flaking and allow medication from your shampoo to work even better. She suggests layering oils with steroid drops as another solution. In this tiered approach, a mild medicated shampoo is alternated with a more medicated shampoo as well as some oils and steroid drops a couple of times a week or when stress levels are high. If you don't love the smell, alternate a medicated shampoo with your regular shampoo or use a regular conditioner.

In fact, many products that are used on the scalp for itching and flaking are topical steroids, and these days they come in the form of mousses or alcohol-based gels. One of the newest solutions on the market is another drug called Luxiq, which is available in a foam or mousse delivery system and can be used day or night. Apply after styling your hair and it will be easily absorbed, which means you can wear a lightweight formula during the day or a greasier version smoothed on before bed so that it works all night. For women who are unwilling to wash their hair more than every two weeks, such as African-American women with braids who want to keep them intact, shampoos won't help; oral and injected steroids are another option. "Some people need steroid injections in the scalp to get deeper into the area that's causing the problem," says Baldwin. "Great for those who can't stand touching their scalp with creams or greasy products, injectable steroids have a deep effect that lasts for a month."

Home Remedies

Try these homemade treatments to maintain a healthy scalp and steer clear of dandruff for good. If they don't work for you, at least they'll add a little extra nourishment to your hair.

- Massage your scalp daily with any of the following ingredients: castor oil or olive oil, castor oil mixed with vinegar, vinegar or lemon juice diluted with an equal amount of water or mint tea, rubbing alcohol, or witch hazel.

- Between shampoos, work cornmeal into your hair and brush it out.

- Before shampooing, rub petroleum jelly or olive oil onto your scalp and cover with a hot, moist towel for 30 minutes.

- Massage a lightly beaten egg (with or without a tablespoon of sea salt) into your dry hair and scalp. Let it permeate for five minutes then rinse and shampoo. If your hair is dry, use egg yolks instead of a whole egg. If your hair is oily but your scalp is dry, substitute an egg white beaten with the juice of a lemon.

- Follow each shampoo with a final rinse of celery seed, rosemary-mint, or wintergreen tea. Add 1 tablespoon of vinegar to increase the benefits. Follow the rinse with a massage of 1 cup apple cider vinegar, 1 tablespoon of witch hazel, and 2 crushed aspirins.

Spa Solutions

Don't trust your beauty skills? Go to a pro. From coast to coast, salons are adding scalp treatments to their menus to keep you ahead of the game when it comes to dandruff.

At New York's Paul Labrecque Salon, try a healthy scalp treatment. First, your scalp will be exfoliated with peppermint essential oil; then lemongrass oil will be applied to the cuticle to close it down, repair damage, and restructure the hair. Hair will feel silkier, smoother, and healthier immediately after the process. A five-week supply of lemongrass can be purchased to continue treatments at home.

At the Los Angeles–based Steam, hair is brushed with a wood-tipped brush to stimulate and revitalize the scalp by bringing the blood flow to the surface and nourish hair follicles and hair strands by bringing natural oils from roots to end. Next, essential oils are applied to the scalp in sections from the top of the head to the nape of the neck, and the neck and shoulders are massaged to help oil rejuvenate the scalp and penetrate the hair shaft. After a rinse and shampoo, the conditioning treatment is applied and hair is steamed for ten minutes to open the cuticle layer and help the conditioner penetrate before the final rinse. Keep in mind that essential oil scalp treatments several times a month will increase blood flow and nourish your hair follicles, so your scalp and hair look their best.

The Scoop on Psoriasis

A chronic genetic condition, psoriasis forms when the skin sheds cells too quickly and they pile up and form thick red scaly patches commonly found on the scalp, elbows, hands, and knees. If the scales stick to the scalp, you may have psoriasis. According to Maria Darnell, director of information services for Hill Dermaceuticals, the makers of Derma-Smoothe FS, psoriasis first manifests itself on the scalp, drying it out and causing crust and scales to form over the pores through which the hair grows. "It basically forms a helmet over the hair follicle and starts to weaken it," says Darnell, who says that although it may spread to other parts of the body, once psoriasis is found on the scalp, it will always remain on the scalp. "You can learn to treat and control, it but you will always have it," she adds. "Your body may go into remission or learn how to manage it more effectively."

"Psoriasis results from inheriting the wrong genes from your parents," says Mark Lebwohl, professor and chairman of the department of dermatology at Mount Sinai School of Medicine, who adds that the disease is also affected by environmental factors including stress and is more common in cold climates than warmer ones. "Characterized by sharply demarcated areas of scaling in the scalp, psoriasis can be treated with a number of different agents, such as shampoos with steroids, fungal preparations like ketoconazole and salicylic acid, which eat away at the scales, or tar, which suppresses inflammation in the scalp." Liquid solutions can be difficult to apply and messy, so most popular treatments come in the form of gels, solutions, lotions, or foams that target the scales and the inflammation.

"Many products designed to treat psoriasis offer strong doses of steroids, only it's not a matter of how strong a steroid is but how well it's delivered and whether or not the area is exposed long enough to reduce inflammation," says Darnell, and cites the oil-based Derma-Smoothe as an example. After a thin layer is applied to a wet scalp, massaged gently, and left overnight, the scales start to loosen and soften. A few hours later, the oil can be washed off with a gentle, nonmedicated shampoo and the scales begin to fall off, allowing the steroid to penetrate the scalp so that hair can grow in healthy again.

Retinoid cream may help for mild cases. For more severe cases, doctors recommend UV light therapy, cortisone creams, coal tar shampoos, antihistamines for itching, PUVA (a medication called psoralen in conjunction with UV light therapy), Accutane, Dovonex, or other prescription meds. Mud from the Dead Sea, rich in potassium chloride, calcium, and magnesium chloride, is also said to help psoriasis.

Recent innovations include olux clobetsol propionate and luxique betamethasone valerate, which turn to liquid when they reach the body's surface temperature. According to Dr. Lebwohl, corticol steroids and other topical preparations are also recommended.

Physician Prescriptions

"If you're using an over-the-counter medicated shampoo and it's not controlling your dandruff—for example, if you still see flaking on your shoulders and you find yourself itching all the time—see your dermatologist," advises Lewis. "Your doctor can determine exactly what the problem is by taking a family history or looking at other parts of your body like your elbows, knees, between your eyebrows or on your nasal folds for similar reactions, including dryness, flaking, and scaling," Baldwin agrees. "If you're using pyrithinone zinc and it's not working, I wouldn't bother with any other active ingredients. Go directly to your dermatologist." Do so before the chain of reactions starts to unfold. Baldwin continues, "If you have bleeding or pus on the scalp, some people get carried away with scratching and get secondarily effected. They can even scratch enough to make the lymph nodes swell and cause an infection, so it's no wonder shampoo stings when you put it on."

If you don't ask for help, you could be in serious trouble. "Some women come in in tears, while others have given up," says Baldwin. "Occasionally, we'll see someone with a bad scalp who has come in with another problem and won't mention the scalp issue. When it's finally addressed, she will say she's used everything and nothing has worked. Women can get incredibly distraught, when, if treated correctly, many scalp problems can be controlled quickly—two or three days to stop the itch and about a week to get rid of the flakes."

Scalp problems like dandruff and psoriasis can be irritating, but at least there are plenty of treatment options. Never underestimate the importance of maintaining a healthy scalp. Suddenly, something as innocuous as going gray doesn't seem like such a big deal in comparison, does it? If you're beginning to notice a bit more salt than pepper in your locks, this may just be your chance to enter this new phase of your life with a whole new shade!

Chapter 9

Graying and Other Color Issues

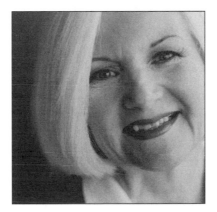

Forget pretty in pink; some women want to be gorgeous in gray. Take these famous females who have made their mark despite their colorless coifs. Fashion model Carmen has been gray for years and still manages to stay professionally booked. Phyllis Diller keeps us in stitches despite her all-gray 'do. Elizabeth Taylor continues to turn heads with her radiant shade of silver. A full head of gray hair didn't stop Dame Judy Dench from walking away with the Oscar for best supporting actress in *Shakespeare in Love*. And just as nonpigmented as gray, former first lady Barbara Bush is known for her signature pearls as well as her snow-white coif.

Say "Nay" to Gray

While a rare handful of women proudly take center stage with their gorgeous gray locks, most others make it their business to keep their grayness well under wraps. Does gray hair make an actress less marketable, an anchorwoman less hirable, a magazine editor less qualified? Why is there such a stigma about gray hair, and what are women doing to avoid falling into the too-bad-she's-gray trap? These are just some of the questions women face as they begin to see their hair turning a grayer shade, usually in their thirties but often as early as their twenties. By age fifty, most women will find that half of their hair will be gray.

Gray Before Your Day

"Graying is a cosmetic problem and can be treated by permanent or temporary hair coloring or by embracing your individuality," says Suzanne Friedler, M.D., a dermatologist with a private practice in New York City. "In some cultures, gray hair is revered as a sign of intelligence and distinction." According to Friedler, the graying of hair is a normal sign of aging and your genes determine how early or late this process begins. A look at your family tree may provide the biggest clue. "Nearly 25 percent of individuals between the ages of twenty-four and thirty-five show signs of graying, and this number increases to 50 percent by the age of fifty," says Friedler. She adds that some people believe that hair can turn gray overnight, but this is not true. "What's actually happening is a form of alopecia areata," she says. "Pig-

Add a Little Spice to Your Life

Some people refer to sprinkles of gray hair as a "salt and pepper" look, which is obviously just a figure of speech. However, a special Japanese pepper called sancho (used in cooking) is being investigated for its ability to rev up the pigmentation cells that control the color of your hair. It is possible, some believe, that sancho pepper may eliminate gray hair permanently.

mented hairs are rapidly lost and white hairs grow in their place, giving the illusion of premature graying." This is a temporary condition and can be treated by a dermatologist. One thing to keep in mind is that early graying (or balding, for that matter) is not a sign of early aging. Despite some reports, no solid link has been found. In general, however, the appearance of a gray hair or two, or more, is simply a sign that you're aging normally.

Still, no matter what the books say, gray hair, like wrinkles, is associated with age. Most women are extremely tempted to pull out their first few gray hairs to remove signs of aging, but this will only distort the hair follicle, resulting in more crinkly hair, which looks coarser. Although some experts argue that gray hair is not coarser but finer. It is, however, drier because the oil glands function less and may create the illusion of coarseness. Some may think brunettes turn gray earlier than others, but that's merely because gray hairs are more prominent on darker heads. It's more difficult to recognize blondes who are turning gray because of the subtler blending of white and gray strands. Adds Friedler, "Graying is more obvious in darker colored hair because of the contrast, but it tends to occur earlier in lighter colored hair, which has a

Vitamin Gray

Scientists believe the intake of certain vitamins is one way of restoring gray hair to its natural color or changing one color to another. The suggested anti-gray vitamins include PABA (para-aminobenzoic acid), calcium pantothenate, choline, and inositol. Try these vitamins in a strong B-complex base and make sure you consume a fair share of milk, brewer's yeast, whole wheat, whole rye, shellfish such as oysters, clams, and shrimp, and meat such as lean pork and ham. Some nutritionists recommend drinking a mixture of two tablespoons each of apple cider vinegar, uncooked honey, and blackstrap molasses in a glass of water every morning.

decreased amount of the enzyme needed to produce melanin so it may gray faster."

Why Gray?

Gray hair has the same structure as pigmented hair but has a hollow core called the medulla, which makes it harder to bend, stiffer, and less manageable.

Melanin contains metals and minerals like iron, zinc, and magnesium, which are oxidative catalysts. Without them, nonpigmented hair develops less oxidative color than pigmented hair, so it's more difficult to color. What's more, gray hair lacks the protective effects of melanin, so it weathers faster when exposed to sunlight and changes natural or applied color.

A few diseases can cause premature graying, including diabetes, pernicious anemia, or thyroid problems. Going into shock or undergoing chemotherapy may cause hair to gray, too. For the most part, though, turning gray is an inherited trait. With genetics playing such a major role, if your mom turned gray early, chances are you will, too. Another genetic factor is the rare occurrence of piebaldism, a condition in which a section or streak of hair is non-pigmented or gray. In actuality, there is no such thing as gray hair. In certain hair follicles, the melanocytes are turned off, which means that melanin, which tints hair, stops being produced and the hair turns white. This is the color of the protein the hair is made of. Therefore, gray hair

Losing Your Gray Naturally

To turn gray hair to dark hair using natural ingredients, experts suggest creating a rinse with dried or fresh sage leaves. It will darken gray hair when added to shampoo or when used as a rinse. Create a strong infusion of at least 4 tablespoons of leaves to a pint of boiling water. Let it sit for several hours or overnight. Strain the liquid from the leaves and rinse hair with the brew. To create a concoction that will last longer, combine a pint of dark sage tea, a pint of bay rum, and an ounce of glycerin. Bottle and label, and apply to hair until it reaches the desired color.

is really a combination of normally pigmented hairs interspersed with white ones.

"Generally, hair sheds constantly each day," says Megan Gordon, owner and head colorist at New York's TwoDo salon, who turned prematurely gray in her teens. "Eventually, the hair follicles stop producing melanin, so you shed brown or blond hairs, then white hairs come in in their place." While it's difficult to determine why this happens, there are several factors that may contribute. For one thing, certain drugs, herbs, and supplements—including vitamin E and echinacea—are known to cause graying. In addition, smoking has been linked to early graying. A study published in the December 21, 1996, issue of the *British Medical Journal* suggests a connection between smoking and gray hair (as well as between smoking and male baldness). The researchers were not, however, able to determine a direct cause-and-effect relationship. People who smoke are four times more likely to be prematurely gray. Some evidence links smoking to early baldness, too. Nutritional problems, such as vitamin B12 deficiency and anemia, can cause grayness, as can thyroid problems and gout. Stress is another gray hair culprit. According to International Trichologist's Philip Kingsley, we know that stress depletes our vitamin B levels. Some studies show that when vitamin B is taken in large doses, the process of graying will begin to be reversed within three months. The hairs revert to white when the vitamins are discontinued.

"Vitamin B may slow down the graying process, but it doesn't get the color back once hair turns gray," says Kingsley, who claims that gene modification, which will introduce a gene that stops hair from turning gray, is still ten years off.

Hormonal levels have an effect on gray hair, too, especially since most women can have at least half a head of gray hair by menopause. That's because when estrogen levels decline at the onset of menopause, cells in the hair follicle begin to multiply more slowly than before, slowing down the regrowth of hair. This process also reduces the production of sebaceous oil and pigment, making the hair finer, sparser, and grayer.

Gray hair should be handled in the same way as naturally pigmented hair, with a few extra precautions. First, it's important to wash and condition gray hair daily. If any type of hair needs frequent shampooing, it's gray hair, as it shows the dirt most of all. Second, gray hair can turn yellow as a result of exposure to several discoloring factors, such as smoke, perms, pollution, sun, mineral deposits, and product buildup. Specially formulated shampoos or rinses with blue or indigo tints are designed to camouflage this yellow tinge. Use them alone until you get the yellow out, then alternate with your regular shampoo. Gray hair can also be conditioned without getting weighed down, which means that regular conditioning can keep the gray shiny and frizz-free.

Keeping Gray at Bay

Coloring gray hair is a little trickier than mixing the chemicals and slapping on the dye. There are several cautions that must be taken to achieve the proper results. "Gray hair is missing the yellow or blue pigments that natural hair would have, so if you just add color, your hair will turn really orange or yellow gold,"

Not All Gray Hair Is Created Equal

If you have oily hair: You'll be tempted to wash your hair more frequently. Keep in mind that each washing strips oil, so it is very important to look for a moisturizing shampoo and conditioner.

If you have dry hair: While you may be able to wash your hair less often, stripping away oil is still a big problem. Conditioning is essential. Consider a leave-in conditioner and a monthly deep-conditioning treatment.

If you have wiry hair: Use a moisturizing shampoo to help put the moisture back into the strands and be sure to avoid any products containing alcohol. Don't forget to condition your hair well. Blow-drying your hair straight with the use of a straightening balm will also help tame the wiry strands.

says Gordon, who suggests adding a large percentage of a natural tone to achieve any color. For example, she says, if more than half of your hair is gray, and you want to color it auburn, mix a blond shade with an auburn tone to make the final result appear natural. Says Gordon, "If your hair is less than 50 percent gray, you have more flexibility in what shade you can choose and in the way you apply it." Gordon, who says that about 90 percent of women color their hair before they turn completely gray, advises deciding how much maintenance you want to invest before you proceed. "Hair-painting and low-lighting require the shortest length of time between visits, about every two to three weeks," she says. "The texture has a lot to do with it. If you have curly hair, the roots won't show as much. Or, you can create more fullness at the root or play with the part to hide the area where the color is growing out."

"Most color lines carry a special series with double pigment in it to cover gray hair, which needs help absorbing color since there is no depth to it," says Amanda Jorge at Prive Salon in Los Angeles. "Women with very light hair in front should have their colorist soften their hair with bleach, then add color. Pre-softening helps hair take color." To get gray coverage, adds Jorge, it is necessary to add neutral colors and a natural base. "If you use straight color, hair will turn red or purple or some other fashion color rather than a believable color, since you will be adding color to hair that has no pigment at all."

MYTH: Hair can turn white overnight.

FACT: Only in your dreams! Your hair is genetically formed and can only be changed with bleach or hair color.

To avoid the expense and the inconvenience of getting an appointment at a salon, most women forgo seeing a pro and opt to color their hair at home. The trick is to do it right to avoid costly color-correcting visits to the hair salon. For best results, color gray hair with vegetable, semi-, or demipermanent color. Keep in mind that the biggest mistakes women make, according to Gordon, are going too dark, going too light, and not adding a natural shade into the formula. Gordon suggests choosing a color that matches your natural shade and another target color. "Generally, anything above medium blond, such as light and lightest blond, won't have enough pigment to cover gray hair," she says. "Medium- to thicker-textured hair would still look gray." Application, she notes, is extremely important. "When coloring gray hair, it's important to be precise in how you apply the color. If you miss a section, you will end up with a white patch." Her general rule of thumb: If your hair is more than 5 percent gray, go to the lightest shade you can carry, so the line of separation as the roots grow in won't be as severe. If you want to maintain a brown background, put in highlights to break up the regrowth line by adding foils across the part and making the highlights two shades lighter.

MYTH: Pull out one gray hair and two will grow.

FACT: The action of pulling out a hair can rupture the follicle and the replacement hair, which will eventually grow, takes longer to regenerate. During this time, another mostly gray hair is beginning to grow next to it. When the hair that you initially pulled out regrows, you will have two gray hairs.

A Head with Red

It takes a special personality to be a redhead. One look at comedy queen Lucille Ball says it all. These days, starlets such as Nicole Kidman, Bernadette Peters, even Sarah Ferguson show us why red is far from dead. No matter how much you want to go red, keep in mind that coloring your hair red is a challenge. For one thing, choosing the right shade is difficult.

Brunettes have natural red tones and can opt for lighter shades of red to emphasize them and still obtain natural-looking results. Red is also difficult to maintain because it's an unstable color and oxidizes more quickly than blond. To keep your red in vivid color, use color-enhancing shampoo and get a gloss treatment at your local salon to seal in color.

Think Pink

Now and again, more radical colors hit the runways and the music video scene and even make their way onto the streets. Take a cue from some of pop's prettiest players who are in the pink, like Lil' Kim, Shakira, Gwen Stefani, and Pink herself. More popular among teenagers and women who yearn for attention, shades of blue and pink give hair color a jolt.

"This re-emerging trend is a flashback from the Eighties," says colorist Doug MacIntosh of Joseph Martin salon. "When placed next to bleached-out hair, pink pieces add texture and pizzazz. The trick to such bold color is that pink streaks can't be retouched without the colors bleeding together, so have fun with it until it grows out."

When it comes to application, MacIntosh advises going to a pro because of the complexity of the process and the risk of dying your skin. If you decide to be daring and do it yourself, remember three things: Wear plastic gloves, put Vaseline around your hairline to keep the dye from adhering to your skin, and have a friend help you.

To create your pink look, the first step is to bleach hair out. Make sure that the bleach you buy is marked "on the scalp" bleach for safety. Other bleaches can cause skin to blister and, believe it or not, your throat to close, leading to serious complications. Divide hair to be dyed light into sections and clip each part away from the rest of your hair. Hair shouldn't be dyed white but pale yellow, to avoid washout. Once the first process is complete, wash hair (don't condition), and blow-dry. Pour on the pink and cover tresses with a plastic cap. Blow-dry again and let color sit for 35 to 45 minutes to allow for full penetration. If you have a bonnet dryer, sit under it with no cap for about an hour, or until hair is fully dry.

Part Three

Hair Thinning & Loss

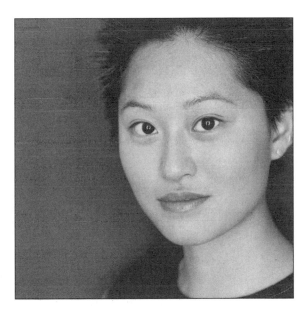

Chapter 10

What Is Hair Loss?

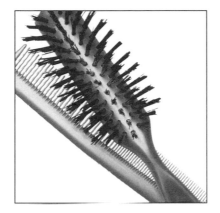

Twenty million women suffer a significant amount of hair loss; about 25 percent show some signs by age forty, but 60 percent of all women experience hair loss by menopause. Gradual loss of hair, as a disease, is a result of alopecia areata or hereditary and aging pattern baldness. Hereditary hair loss is caused by a gradual miniaturization of certain hair follicles, which makes hair grow in shorter and thinner and eventually stop growing.

Think you're thinning? Different women grow and shed hair at different rates. At any given time, as much as 85 percent of the scalp hair is growing up to an inch a month and may continue to grow for two to six

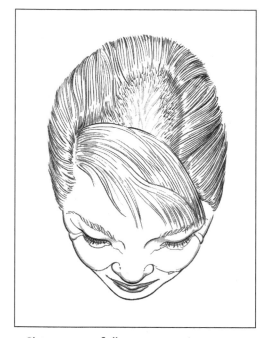

Sixty percent of all women experience some hair loss by menopause. Twenty-five percent show signs of hair loss by age forty.

years without stopping. When the phase ends, each hair has a two- to six- month resting period and then begins a shedding phase. Only 10 to 15 percent of hair is in the resting phase at one time. Before long, a new strand of hair begins to sprout from the root, replacing the older strand above it, thus a new growth period begins. New hair can grow back shorter and thinner in diameter, so it takes up less space on your scalp. Experts remind us that it's normal to shed 50 to 100 hairs a day and not likely to be noticeable, since most of us have 100,000 hairs on our head.

What's Your Hair Problem?

Most types of hair loss are often diagnosed as hereditary. After all, now that we know most women will suffer some sort of hair loss as they age, we can always chalk it up to our genetic predispositions. Women are born with androgens, the male hormones that cause hair loss if you are genetically predisposed, as well as estrogens, the female hormones that have the opposite effect.

"Whenever the hormone testosterone is present, there is a possibility of female androgenic alopecia," explains Shelley Friedman, D.O., president of the American Board of Hair Restoration Surgery. "Testosterone has an opportunity to change into a bad hormone called dihydrotestosterone, which can cause hair loss. The enzyme 5-alpha reductase is the catalyst that turns testosterone into dihydrotestosterone, so until your body has access to it, which is usually when you hit adolescence, you won't experience hair loss. "We all have 5-alpha reductase, but the follicles in the scalp can either be sensitive or insensitive to dihydrotestosterone. The degree of hair loss that we experience is dependent on which of our follicles are sensitive. Women with hair follicles that are sensitive to dihydrotestosterone will have a receding hairline. Those with sensitive follicles in the crown region will have a bald spot at the back of their head. It's all genetic."

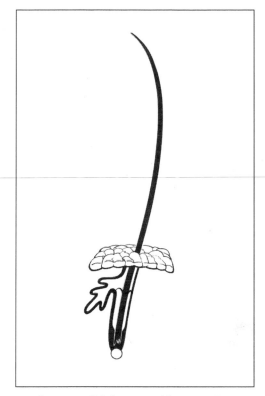

As we age, hair becomes thinner, starting at the root. At around age forty, follicle size begins to narrow.

Female pattern baldness occurs when hair falls out but new hair does not grow in its place. This problem is associated with genetic predisposition, aging, and levels of endocrine hormones or androgens. Changes in the levels of the androgens can affect hair production. For example, after the hormonal changes of menopause, many women find that the hair on their head has thinned, while facial hair becomes coarser. Although new hair is not produced, the follicle remains alive, suggesting the possibility of new hair growth. Unlike male pattern baldness, in female pattern baldness, hair thins all over the head, but the frontal hairline is maintained. There may be a moderate loss of hair on the crown, but this will rarely result in complete baldness. A skin biopsy or other procedure may be used to diagnose medical disorders that cause loss of hair.

Most women don't mind baring their souls but have a big problem baring their scalp. Unfortunately, though usually mild to moderate, female pattern baldness is permanent. The only drug or medication approved by the United States Food and Drug Administration (FDA) to treat female pattern baldness is minoxidil (Rogaine), used topically on the scalp, which we will discuss further in Chapter 12. Hair loss recurs when usage is stopped.

Are You a Loser? Early Symptoms and Warning Signs

Thinning hair is a natural part of aging. Even women who are considerably healthy have hair that is thickest at age twenty and it begins to thin thereafter. That's why it's important to be prepared for our hair to thin, so that we can recognize the signs at an early stage and slow the process while we still have plenty of hair on our heads. Try these simple tests to determine if you are starting to lose your hair.

- Check your pillow, hairbrush, and the shower drain, or run your hand through wet hair, for excessive shedding.

- Check the width of your part. If you see a wider part than normal, that means that there is a greater amount of space between each hair and you are probably experiencing hair loss or androgenetic alopecia.

- Measure the diameter of your ponytail to see if it has become smaller. Place your thumb and forefinger around your hair in ponytail formation. Close your fingers firmly until they hold your hair. If they form a dime-size circle or smaller, your hair is thin. If they form a quarter-size circle or larger, the hair strand is considered thick.

- In the scalp region, try to identify shorter, thinner, less pigmented hairs with pointy ends.

- Ask yourself if you've recently changed your daily routine by incorporating crash diets, oral contraceptives, or other medications.

Any of these tests will help you determine whether you need to see a dermatologist or a specialized stylist for advice.

Two percent of the population at one time or another suffers from alopecia areata, an extensive condition in which hair loss occurs in noticeable bald patches. It can be evident in one large patch or many small ones. What is actually happening is that when the hair grows, it appears white in the center and regains color as it gets longer. One of the most common forms is complete loss of hair on the head in a circular patch 1–10 cm in diameter.

Alopecia totalis, a severe form of alopecia areata, is characterized by a complete loss of scalp hair and is caused by the body's attack on normal hair follicles. Hair suddenly falls out in a generalized pattern, resulting in complete baldness of the scalp.

Other common types of hair loss include:

- Cicatricial alopecia, an irreversible form of hair loss associated with scarring, usually on the scalp.

- Congenital alopecia is the congenital absence of scalp hair, which may occur alone or be part of a more widespread disorder.

- Friction alopecia, a result of wearing snug-fitting wigs or hats, is a form of hair loss that can easily be remedied.

- Symptomatic alopecia, the loss of hair due to systemic or psychogenic causes, such as general ill health, infections of the scalp or skin, nervousness, a specific disease such as typhoid fever, or stress. The hair may fall out in patches, or there may be diffused loss of hair instead of complete baldness in one area.

- Traction alopecia, the loss of hair caused by ponytails, braids, or cornrows that are pulled too tight, yanking hair out by its roots.

- Anogen effluvian is the loss of hair that occurs when undergoing chemotherapy. In this condition, all growing hairs fall out.

- Telogen effluvian, generalized hair shedding, often occurs after an acute illness or pregnancy. It's normal for adults to lose between 75 to 100 hairs a day, but certain instances can cause an increase in hair loss by inducing hair follicles to reenter the telogen (resting) phase. About 95 percent of women develop some degree of hair loss after giving birth or stopping birth control pills. Other causes include high fever, surgery, psychiatric stress, bulimia, dieting, and malnutrition. New hair will replace those that fall out.

Common Myths

Scientists have been studying the life cycle of hair for years. Biologists understand much about the development of our hair follicles from their first embryonic appearance to the last stages of life. Proteins play a role in directing many of those steps, and researchers are uncovering additional "regulatory" molecules as well. Yet despite new developments, there is still much to learn about why hair begins to thin and fall out.

MYTH: Shaving one's head will cause hair to grow back thicker.

FACT: Shaving one's head will result in . . . a shaved head! Triggered by stress, hair that is lost in alopecia areata will sometimes grow back after the stress disappears. In other cases, treatment is necessary. Complete baldness is rare. The psychological damage associated with alopecia areata is the most damaging aspect of the condition since it is sudden and unexpected. Alopecia areata tends to appear in families with a history of asthma, eczema, or autoimmune disorders, such as rheumatoid arthritis or lupus erythematosus. It can be treated with cortisone injections, topical minoxidil (Rogaine), or other medications that stimulate hair growth.

One of the biggest misconceptions is that only 15 to 20 percent of women experience hair thinning, when in fact 50 percent of women will experience some degree of thinning by age fifty; virtually all of us will experience thinning after age fifty. In addition, while many women think hair thinning always begins in women in their 50s, 60s, or 70s, thinning in women actually occurs in their 20s, 30s, or 40s. And though women may experience hair thinning just as men do, they can also lose their hair in a completely different way. Unlike men, who get bald spots, women experience diffused thinning, particularly in the crown and temporal areas of the scalp, which is often easier to camouflage.

Many women who experience male pattern baldness believe it is inherited from their mother's side of the family. The fact is, the gene for male pattern baldness can come from the mother's or father's gene pool.

Therefore, baldness can be inherited from either side of the family since many genes can be involved. So there's no point in studying your family history and paying close attention to how soon your mom's or dad's hair falls out. Your hair loss process is entirely unique to you.

All women lose hair at some point during the day, whether it's while brushing, combing, washing, or styling their hair, or whether their hair falls out on their pillow while they are sleeping or into the drain while they are in the shower. Sometimes women lose over 100 hairs per day, and many times they don't even notice, or they are aware of the loss but think it's normal. If you don't have male pattern baldness, new hairs will soon replace the hairs that fall out. If you do have male pattern baldness, however, even losing the "normal" 75 to 150 hairs a day can be a concern, because many of those hairs are being shed by follicles that are in the process of dying. Therefore, the new hairs those follicles create will be progressively thinner, until the follicles are only capable of making fine peach-fuzz hairs. Eventually, those follicles will die and no longer produce any hairs at all.

So you're losing your hair. You may think that all you have to do is eat right, exercise, or start a religious Rogaine regimen to increase the number of hair follicles on your head. But while a proper diet and a healthy workout routine will do your body good, they won't help add to the number of follicles you have. Actually, the number and diameter of your hair follicles are a hereditary issue and completely out of your control. Nothing you do will alter how many hair follicles you have. You can, however, use preventative and treatment measures outlined in this book to combat the follicle-killing effect of DHT, the androgen created when the hormone testosterone is acted upon by the enzyme 5-alpha-reductase.

Another known misconception is the belief that hair will keep growing and growing if you never get it cut. Even if you've always wondered what your hair would look like at its longest, the truth is that the length of your hair depends on its natural cycle, which is unique to each individual. The longer the hair's growth phase, the longer the hair will grow. If you have a naturally long growth phase, you can grow your hair to well below your waist. If you have a naturally shorter growth phase, your hair will be shed before it grows that long and will only grow to a certain length. The duration of your particular growth phase is based on heredity and is affected by nutrition.

Healthy diets are always helpful in maintaining hair that's strong and beautiful. In Chapter 13 of this book, we discuss natural and nutritional treatments for hair loss as well as foods and dietary vitamins and supplements that can help hair stay healthy and looking beautiful. Does this mean you can chow down on a meal of steak and potatoes every night? Or do you have to maintain a strict diet of fruits, vegetables, and proteins to keep hair looking great? There is a connection between balding and eating animal fat, particularly red meat, because high-fat diets lead to greater DHT production and more damage to hair follicles. But it's a good idea to maintain a well-balanced diet, with a healthy portion of all of the necessary good groups.

If you haven't worn a hat in years because you think it may have an effect on hair loss, it's time to rummage through the closet for your favorite topper and get back into the swing of covering your head. Surprisingly enough, many women believe that wearing a hat causes hair loss. But it's just not true. Experts believe that as long as you don't wear a hat that's so tight it restricts circulation-blood flow to the hair follicles, it will not cause hair loss. Hats can, however, damage hair because of the effects of sweat, dirt, and skin particles that can clog pores. So make sure the inside of your hat is kept scrupulously clean. Blow-drying your hair does not cause hair loss, but excessive heat and intensive styling can damage hair. It can dry, burn, and fray hair that may then fall out, to be replaced by new hair that will sprout from the follicle beneath the skin during the growth phase. Curling and straightening irons can have a similar effect, so keep styling with them to a minimum. If you're hanging around the house all day on a Saturday, give your hair a break and skip the styling process. Or let hair air-dry every other day during the week to give it a break from the harmful effects of the heat that comes along with some of the best-looking styles.

Some women go a couple of days in between shampoos because they believe frequent shampooing will make their hair fall out faster and in greater excess. If you are afraid to shampoo your hair in the shower because you see so much hair coming out in the drain, know that everyone loses a certain amount of hair when it's wet. You may actually think you notice it more in the shower when you have to clean it out of the drain or on your bathroom floor, which is usually not carpeted and a good backdrop for hair to show up on. Shampooing only loosens the hair follicle's base and may actually cause faster growth as the massage action of shampooing has a stimulating effect on hair.

No woman is exempt from the problem of hair loss. The rumor that hair loss only happens to Caucasian women with fine, blond hair is just that: a rumor. While it's true that women with fine hair are more likely to experience thinning, it is also true that hair may thin regardless of its texture—and thinning has nothing to do with hair color or ethnicity. In fact, African-American women account for a large portion of the consumers who seek out hair loss remedies, products, and treatments. Asian women also experience thinning and other hair problems at high rates. High levels of stress can also cause temporary hair loss. Anxiety and tension have no lasting effect on the condition of the hair. Once the problem is treated, thinning will stop and eventually hair will grow. There is also a lot of debate about whether or not hair loss is seasonal. Some people believe hair grows most in the spring when testosterone levels are lowest, and hair loss accelerates in the fall when testosterone levels peak. Others go so far as to say that twice as much hair is lost in the fall as in the spring. But we know that the bottom line is that everyone loses hair according to her own time schedule. There is no hard-and-fast season-related rule that applies.

Although there is some comfort in knowing that many of the common myths associated with hair loss are far from factual, the reality is that many women do encounter some degree of hair thinning. And, when they do, it can be an extremely difficult and emotional experience. Psychological stress and a loss of self-esteem can be an issue for many women, in reaction to their change in appearance.

Chapter 11

The Emotional Effects
of Hair Loss

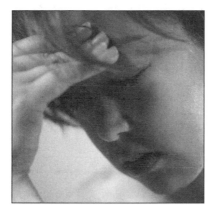

One of the most distressing factors on the list of unpleasant side effects for cancer patients is hair loss. For some women, whose regular salon visits are a part of a whole well-honed grooming routine, the news that hair loss could be imminent is a nasty shock. Other women who may not suffer from the disease but suddenly find themselves losing hair can also suffer embarrassment, humility, and lack of self-esteem.

A recent study by the Women's Institute for Fine and Thinning Hair shows that women with thinning hair feel less feminine, less likely to succeed professionally, embarrassed, helpless, less desirable to men, socially unacceptable, and less sexy, making it difficult for them to cope with every-day life. But thanks to psychological experts, support groups, and salon pro-grams designed to meet their specific needs, women who are undergoing the loss of their hair have new hope and a brighter outlook.

MYTH: Stress causes permanent hair loss.

FACT: Although it's true that stress can be a factor in the temporary thinning of hair, it has no lasting effect on the condition of the hair. Once stress is treated, thinning no longer occurs as a symptom of that condition.

Coming to Terms

"While losing your hair may not be as dramatic or traumatic as los-ing a breast, the effects can be almost as far-reaching in terms of self-image," says Rachel Schultz, a psychotherapist, based in New Jersey, spe-cializing in women's issues. "Hair has always been called the crowning glory, the flowing tresses, the hallmark of femininity. When we start to lose it, we can see how it affects our self-image and sense of self as a woman." To put the problem in perspective, Schultz suggests directing the focus on the things about yourself that you value beyond your physical image, such as your career and your role in your family. And, she says, just because you are losing your hair doesn't mean you still can't be sexual and attractive. "It's important to continue to wear makeup, work out, keep yourself in shape, and focus on who you are and what you are inside," she says. "Concentrate on the power and strength you reflect. If you start slip-ping, join a support group that deals with women who are struggling with self-image issues."

Up Your Confidence Level and Boost Your Body Image

Women who are down about losing their hair can have their faith restored by the people who deal with the issues involved every day. "People come to me in tears because their hair is coming out and they have seen doctors who tell them there's nothing they can do about it," says Lynn Glaze, owner of Sheer Reflections in Pineville, Louisiana, a John Paul Mitchell Systems and Rogaine Trainer for the JPMS Color and Professional Scalp Therapy System and a member of the American Cancer Society's team of specialists who help women regain their self-esteem and their stylish appearance after cancer therapy. "I take them through testimonies from other people and show them their successes. We don't have any clients that have been put on the Rogaine regimen that have stopped using it, and having their hairdressers involved works to their advantage."

Glaze points out that hairdressers are among a handful of professionals—which includes doctors—who actually touch people. "When you put your hands on someone, they trust you," she says. "They are open to trying the hair regrowth and volumizing products that a stylist recommends." Surprisingly enough, Glaze says it's more of a challenge to get hairdressers to understand that this is a serious thing. "It doesn't matter what someone else sees, it's how you feel about yourself."

Through Paul Mitchell's scalp therapy system, clients are encouraged to use shampoo and conditioner even after the first shampoo, during which time oil and debris on the scalp is removed. The hair regrowth and volumizing products should also be used in your daily hair care regime, and within a month, you will see half an inch of new growth. "It's true, look in the mirror," says Glaze. "There will be tiny strands of hair that aren't long enough to lay over yet, but there will be a lot of growth going on." One of the hardest things about treating thinning hair is to recognize that it's happening to you and practice preventative maintenance prior to the actual hair loss. "A bit of excess hair loss is normal," says Glaze. "But if you notice a good amount of hair in the drain after you shampoo, or after you run your fingers through it when it's wet, you should be addressing the issue. Instead, many women are embarrassed about it and come into the salon under the pretense of getting a haircut." Glaze advises trying Paul Mitchell's Botanical Hydrating shampoo, which provides body building for fine, thinning, or color-treated hair and Botanical Body Building Rinse detangler for fine, thinning hair. Paul Mitchell products also use thermal strengthening therapy to heat up and increase the circulation on the scalp and come packaged in a kit with Rogaine (2 percent Monoxil for women, 5 percent for men).

Tress Stress

For many women, hair loss is a stress-related issue. Schultz advises using various stress-management techniques to control your stress level and bring your rate of hair growth back to normal. According to Schultz, deep breathing is key. "Focus on the center of the body and the diaphragm and breath very deeply," she says. "Next, try visualizations. Close your eyes and picture yourself in a calm, serene place like a park or at the ocean and think of this image all the time. After the first few times, you will find a combination that works for you, whether it includes breathing, visualizations, music, even knitting, or anything else that you've found de-stresses you." If stress isn't the problem, maybe there are psychotherapy issues to deal with. Try to incorporate cognitive behavioral techniques that make you feel better about yourself. Keep telling yourself that you are beautiful, strong, and worthy. Says Schultz, "If you say it enough and internalize it, you'll believe it."

At the Avon salon in New York City, hair care and styling advice comes completely free for cancer patients. Senior stylist Joelle has pioneered the Breast Cancer Awareness Support Program, after being inspired by two sisters who were diagnosed the same week with different cancers. The sisters subsequently had very different hair needs—one wore a wig, one did not. After carefully and sensitively helping them through their individually tailored hair treatments, Joelle decided to devote every Wednesday afternoon from 5:00 P.M. to 7:00 P.M. to cancer patients and all their hair needs.

"My goal is to be a friend and a support system," she says. "Most medics can't gauge how much hair you will lose when you undergo chemotherapy, so first it's about bending to patients' needs. It can be pretty traumatic losing any hair and there are ways to overcome it. If hair falls out sufficiently to warrant needing a wig, I suggest patients buy two. We can cut one to their own hair length and the other to a shorter style, which they wear around the house, while the other is being washed. This gets them used to shorter hairstyles and the regrowth procedure. Also, if they decide after hair is thinning to cut it all off, I never do it in one fell swoop. I patiently take them through a series of haircuts to show how they can look at all differentiating lengths. I don't bring up the word 'wig' until the patient does. Only then do I advise on where to buy and the benefits of human hair or synthetic."

Depression and Hair Loss: Cause or Effect?

Although losing your hair can cause you stress or lead you to become depressed, the reverse is also true: feeling stressed out or depressed can actually lead to hair loss. Depression can cause imbalances in your physical body, affecting your entire endocrine system and causing hair loss as a side effect. According to Mitch Peritz, Washington, D.C.–based chiropractor and nutritionist, "There are many factors that contribute to depression, which all play a role in hair loss. Physiologic factors include the endocrine system and the production and balance of certain hormones, especially cortisol, thyroid hormones, and estrogen. Blood glucose levels are also related to stress and hair loss, as well as specific neurotransmitters, including L-hydroxytryptophan. Cortisol, produced from the adrenal glands, increases

•

or decreases with the amount of stress that a person experiences. Fluctuations in the amount of cortisol, Dehydroepiandrosterone (DHEA), and estrogen can all contribute to hair loss. These are all affected by stress and conditions such as pregnancy and menopause. After menopause, it is important to evaluate DHEA levels because if they are abnormal, the type of estrogen that a woman is taking may have to be changed.

"Decreased amounts of thyroid hormones will also cause hair loss. It is often difficult to determine if a person is hypothyroid. Blood tests are not always accurate and many different lab tests may have to be performed. Serial body temperature measurements as well as iodine absorption tests may help diagnose hypothyroidism. Other clinical signs include depression, headaches, cold extremities, dry hair and skin problems, and gastrointestinal abnormalities. Queen Anne's sign is the name of a condition that causes a person to lose the lateral third part of the eyebrow, and this is often a diagnostic for hypothyroidism.

"Optimal organ function is also crucial for hair homeostasis. Certain diseases and conditions—or even aging—can interfere with the body's ability to produce specific hormones or to eliminate toxins from the body, which can cause depression and hair loss. The proper function of the adrenal glands can influence the utilization and production of the thyroid hormones. The entire endocrine system along with the body's hormones interplay to maintain proper organ function.

"There are other things that can affect the thyroid hormones. Iodine is important for the production of these hormones, and things such as fluoride and chlorine may displace iodine, causing a decrease in the thyroid hormone production. Some people may have to avoid certain toothpastes, tap water, or swimming, if they have sensitivities to these substances. There are also certain foods that interfere with the production of thyroid hormones, including millet grains and cruciferous vegetables such as broccoli, kale, brussel sprouts, and mustard greens."

Styling Secrets

There are plenty of styling tricks for hair that's just starting to thin or fall out. Shampoo with products made with dimethicone and dimethicone copolyol, which build hair volume. Most thickening shampoos are designed to add body and improve texture. If using a thickening shampoo, it's a good idea to condition hair before, to get the benefits of conditioning without weighing hair down. When styling, use a blow dryer at a low setting to add volume to your hair and help point it in the right direction to style. Mousses or gels can make hair look thinner by weighing it down. Instead, use a good root lifter with resin and plant extract to help lift hair at the root without stiffness and a volumizer with panthenol to thicken hair fibers for fuller-looking hair. After drying hair completely, mist hair with a good hair spray or finishing spray, then comb through, and style as you like. The right hair-cut and color can also make a difference. According to Lynn Glaze, cutting a few layers into your otherwise one-level look adds depth and makes hair appear a bit thicker. She shows her clients how to use styling and heat-protective products and illustrates different styling techniques, using round brushes and curling irons while they are in the chair, so they know how to style their hair when they get home. Lightening or highlighting the front of the hair draws attention to those areas and makes the thinning areas less noticeable, especially if you have a drastic contrast between your skin and hair color.

Changes in our physical appearance can have a profound impact on our emotional attitude. And though it's important to acknowledge a loss—even when it's hair—there's no reason to be discouraged. There are many possibilities when it comes to hair replacement—from pharmaceutical and surgical treatments to natural and nutritional remedies.

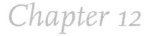

Chapter 12

Medical and Pharmaceutical Treatments

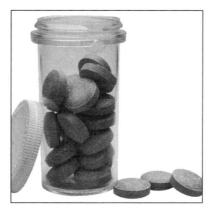

Just when you thought wishing for a full head of hair was about as insane as hoping you would win the lottery, the hair gods indulge you with a handful of medications and products designed to arouse your follicles, urge hair growth, and give you something to smile about at the same time.

Miracle Medications

"Surprisingly enough, it seems that the most effective medications for male baldness or hair loss were discovered by accident," says Marc Klein, RPh, cofounder and CFO of YPRx.com (Your Pharmacist Recommends) and a New York City–based pharmacist. "For example, Rogaine and Propecia are the two best-selling hair loss medications on the market and they were both discovered as side effects of other drugs." Cortisone is another product that was first recognized in the hair growth market as a side effect, since it was originally used mainly for many immune-mediated diseases like lupus and anti-inflammatory conditions, and not primarily used to treat hair loss. Experts will agree, however, that it's not widely marketed for hair loss because it contains steroids and is too dangerous to take long term. Side effects from extensive steroid intake can include increased susceptibility to infection, disruption of electrolyte balances, which may cause hypokalemia (a decrease in potassium in the body), sodium retention, fluid retention, weight gain, and growth suppression in children. Another important effect of steroids in women is the loss of bone mass or osteoporosis. This can cause a dramatic change in a woman's personal and physical appearance. The face can widen and look "fat," among other endocrinological problems.

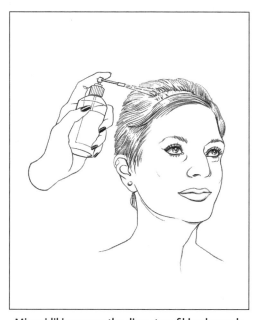

Minoxidil increases the diameter of blood vessels and improves circulation. It is applied topically.

Certain dermatologists who specialize in treating men with hair loss combine Retin-A (tretinoin) with Rogaine (minoxidil) or Lontein (minoxidil) with the hope that the tretinoin will help exfoliate the skin and allow the minoxidil to penetrate deeper into the scalp, causing a more pronounced effect. How they work: Minoxidil is used as a peripheral vasodilator, increasing the diameter of blood vessels and improving circulation. Its hypertensive properties have a direct vasodilating effect on vascular smooth muscle, which causes a decrease in blood pressure.

"Physicians started prescribing minoxidil for various medical conditions and a side effect known as reversible hypertrichosis [elongation, thickening, and enhanced pigmentation of fine body hair] was noticed," explains Shelly Friedman, president of the American Board of Hair Restoration Surgery and a physician who certifies doctors in hair transplantation surgery. "Later it was found out that, if applied topically, minoxidil can cause hair-growth stimulation. The mechanism, however, by which this happens is unknown. Some theories include possibilities that minoxidil may alter androgen metabolism in the scalp, or it may exert a local vasodilation effect, enhancing microcirculation around the hair follicle. Others believe it may directly stimulate the hair follicle." Proscar, which in a lower dose is known as Propecia (finasteride), was originally administered for systematic benign prostatic hyperplasia (BPH), a condition of enlargement of the prostate causing symptoms in older men. According to Friedman, Propecia was originally known to competitively inhibit the steroid 5-alpha-reductase, an enzyme that is responsible for formation of the potent androgen 5-alpha-dihydrotestosterone (DHT) from testosterone. It is DHT that seems to be most responsible for hair loss in men. Because DHT influences the development of the prostate gland, decreasing levels of this hormone, it should relieve the symptoms associated with BPH. One side effect is hirsutism, or hair growth. The manufacturer of Propecia determined that in order to get hair growth, it was important to decrease the strength from 5 mg to 1 mg, which would aid in the treatment of male pattern baldness.

Scary Side Effects

While Rogaine and Propecia are the best products on the market for hair loss, they may stimulate certain side effects in some women. According to Friedman, some people who take Rogaine complain of a red, itchy, dry scalp because of the alcohol content (30 percent alcohol and 50 percent propylene glycol). To treat it, Friedman recommends using a good conditioner every day, and an oil treatment once a week to replace lost moisture on the scalp. He also recommends that women try the 2-percent formulation instead of the 5-percent version, since evidence suggests there are no additional benefits to the higher dosage in women. "In addition to the itching factor, you have to cover the scalp with Rogaine twice a day, indefinitely, for it to work," adds Redmond. "Some women find this process practically difficult to fit into their daily routines." In addition, Rogaine has a heavy, oily texture and putting it on twice a day in the morning hours makes women's hair look and feel oily for the rest of the day. To counteract that, dilute the dosage half and half with water and make sure to apply it to the skin of the scalp, not the hair.

While side effects of Propecia are specifically sexual in men, such as a decreased libido, decreased ejaculate, and sexual dysfunction, the only known drawback for women is that it should definitely be avoided if you are are of childbearing age. The reason for this is that Propecia blocks the production of 5-alpha-reductase, which turns testosterone into dihydrotestosterone. This means there will be an increased amount of testosterone, which can cause birth defects in a male fetus if the woman is pregnant.

Other research shows that postmenopausal women had no response to Propecia, which means women are picking up the 5-alpha-reductase enzyme in some other way or converting testosterone to dihydrotestosterone in another way. This proves that the same medication doesn't react similarly on women as it does on men.

Preventative Products

Some products on the market offer preventative help. "When hair loss is caused by genetics, it's important to try to practice preventative maintenance by using shampoos, conditioners, sprays, gels, and other products that have been proven to stimulate hair growth and stop hair loss," says Lynn Glaze, owner of Sheer Reflections in Pineville, Louisiana, and a John Paul Mitchell Systems and Rogaine trainer. "Paul Mitchell shampoo with mushroom extract helps stimulate hair growth and prevent further hair loss by keeping the hair follicle clean of sebaceous oils that the body excretes and providing a healthy environment for hair to grow."

MYTH: Certain cosmetic products will make hair thicker.

FACT: There are no cosmetic products that have been developed to date that will permanently change hair thickness. However, there are products that will help improve hair texture temporarily and many products offer appropriate and effective solutions under many circumstances.

At the Paul Mitchell Hair Regrowth Center, trained staff members consult clients on recognizing the symptoms of hair thinning or loss and taking actions that will help retard or reverse the process. Says Glaze, "When women come in to the center, we try to find out whether or not they are seeing excess hair in their brush or on their pillow, if they have recently changed their diets, or if they are taking any new medications or hormones. Most of the time they will see hair loss as normal and continue to use the same products." Glaze explains that Pharmacia and Paul Mitchell have joined forces to compile hair regrowth kits that feature Paul Mitchell Scalp Therapy shampoo, conditioner for maintenance, and a bottle of Rogaine to help the user stimulate hair growth. Part of an extensive product line, the shampoo should be used daily and sits on the scalp for three to five minutes to ensure that the extracts get into the hair shaft to provide a clean, healthy environment. Paul Mitchell bodifying gels, sculpting foams, and volumizing sprays are all designed to thicken fine hair. Even Paul Mitchell color products are made with low ammonia to ensure subtle lift of the cuticle layer for stronger hair and so that you don't have the dry feeling of color you can get from other products. Suspended in beeswax to condition hair, they also contain eucalyptus oil for a cooling effect on the scalp. Glaze monitors clients for thirty days and tracks the results.

Hormonal Help

Hormones of all kinds regulate every working mechanism in the body, from body functions to emotions. The body facilitates communication among cells via electrical impulses that travel through nerve fibers called neurons and by chemicals that are carried through the endocrine system, which uses hormones as messengers. The glands of the endocrine system release hormones into the bloodstream, which carries them to all parts of the body. For women, the glands of the endocrine system include the pituitary gland, which is located at the base of the front part of the brain, the thyroid and parathyroid glands, which can be found at the front of the neck, the adrenal glands, which are adjacent to the top of the kidneys with one gland above each kidney, the pancreas, which can be found behind the stomach in the abdominal cavity, and the ovaries in the pelvic area. The hypothalamus is the control center in the brain and regulates basic body function. It controls the pituitary glands, which were created to receive messages about an organ or area's need for a particular hormone and to secrete that hormone or trigger another gland to release its desired hormone.

"Most targeted therapies that are hormonal are topical oil formulations meant to block the conversion of testosterone to dihydrotestosterone and the effects of testosterone on hair follicles and oil glands," says Wilma

F. Bergfeld, head of clinical research, department of dermatology, the Cleveland Clinic in Cleveland, Ohio. "However, nothing is close to being FDA approved." Bergfeld cites anti-androgens such as L-dactone and cyrpodium acetate, a birth control pill with a specific progesterone, as being very effective in reducing the testosterone effect on hair follicles, which allows them to grow longer and bigger.

Androgenic alopecia deals with the male androgen hormone and the genetic component you are born with. "The hormone that causes the hair follicle to become inactive is testosterone," says Geoffrey Redmond, a New York City–based endocrinologist specializing in female hormone problems. With the most extensive experience in the world working with hormonal treatments for hair loss, Redmond explains that estrogen has the opposite effect and keeps the hair on your head longer. "Most women with hair loss have normal levels of testosterone, but hair follicles that are over sensitive to the hormone are usually that way because of genetic reasons. These women will also notice other skin and hair changes, such as oily skin and acne as well as increased facial and body hair."

Hormonal hair loss, according to Redmond, is most noticeable on the crown or top of the head and at the temples. "Unlike men who experience hair recession, women either don't see a recession or only see it slightly," says Redmond. "This confuses doctors who think that if hair loss is hormonal, the hairline will recede, but this isn't necessarily true." Redmond adds that people need to lose a substantial amount of hair to realize they have thinning hair. "Women notice that their hair is thinning before anyone else does because they know their own hair," he says. "Occasionally, the hairdresser notices it, but your doctors can't tell unless it's traumatic. This leads to frustration in women that people in health care don't take them seriously."

Testosterone can also cause more oil to be present in the form of oily hairs or crust on the scalp. This condition isn't caused by hormones, but women who have it have an increased chance of having an underactive thyroid. While it's a serious condition that should be addressed, treating the thyroid doesn't directly help the hair.

Other hormonal factors of hair loss include a lack of estrogen. "Estrogen lengthens the hair cycle and makes hair stay on the head longer, so when levels fall during menopause, the hair doesn't stay in place as long," says Redmond. "This can begin in perimenopause or can start years after menstruation has stopped. When we look at women in their 70s and 80s, we see they have thin hair. Hormonal replacement therapy helps—in fact some women take it only to improve the condition of their hair—but each woman needs a dose that specifically targets her needs." Women have circulating levels of testosterone effects, and as long as estrogen levels are sufficiently high testosterone effects that commonly appear in men, such as hair loss from the breakdown of products of testosterone, are not manifested in women. However, in the perimenopausal period and when menopause finally occurs, estrogen levels drop so testosterone effect that are unopposed and hair thinning and loss can occur more rapidly, as it does in men. One additional benefit of hormone replacement therapy is maintenance of the robust condition of hair and maintenance of the hair cycle.

Follicle Forecast

As in all areas of medicine, there are always new theories to test, new hypotheses to check out. Scientists are currently studying anti-androgens, or drugs that counteract the effect of the male hormone testosterone, which is responsible for signaling hair to fall out. Growth factors are being studied to see if the growth of the tissue of the hair follicle can be encouraged.

Gene therapy, according to Friedman, is a major area of study in the field of hair loss. Through a discovery of a gene linked to a rare form of alopecia, in which people lose all of their hair, scientists were able to conduct experiments to try to determine different ways to grow hair cells. The objective is to try to identify the genes involved in hair growth and hair loss in order to develop the ability to deliver a gene's DNA coding to hair follicles. Using a gunlike instrument, it is now possible to selectively target genes to the most important cells of the hair follicle so, for example, these days there are ways to deliver melanin, which delivers hair color to the hair follicles. "As far as the future is concerned," says Bergfeld, "gene manipulation is being studied as a mechanism of hair promotion. Retardation of hair growth is still being investigated, since we don't totally understand hair follicle regeneration and the growth cycle. Some genes have been identified but not all, so the areas of mechanism and gene influence are under continued investigation. Right now there are only a few people in the country who like to treat hair loss, but there's hope for the future. Innovative surgical treatments like hair transplantation micrographs and scalp reductions, as well as a combination, are in the works."

Increasing the hair's growth cycle with PTH is another focus. According to Friedman, scientists are trying to figure out how to block PTHrP, a chemical that causes the hair follicles to go into the resting cycle, so that hair follicles will return to their growth phase. They are also studying 5-alpha-reductase inhibitors in an attempt to learn how to inhibit the production of the enzyme, which converts testosterone to dihydrotestosterone, which kills hair follicles.

Cycotol, a drug that is used externally as a topical lotion applied to the head, blocks the effects of testosterone on hair follicles. There is also research being done on aromatase, an enzyme that blocks or deactivates the effect of dihydrotestosterone on hair follicles. L'Oréal Pharmaceuticals in Paris has developed a drug that is marketed in France to treat women's androgenetic alopecia. Dercos, which is sold over the counter, combats the hardening of hair follicles, a hair loss–causing condition that's prevalent among women with female pattern baldness.

There are plenty of other studies in the works. According to International Trichologist Philip Kingsley, RU 58841 is an androgen receptor blocker that inhibits the effects of testosterone and DHT on hair follicles. As a result of the effects of baldness from radiation in cancer patients, the National Cancer Institute is studying the effects of topically applying nitroxide radical tempol to the scalp to prevent hair loss. The process of cloning is being studied, so as a patient, you can donate to yourself all of the hair you need regardless of how little hair you may have left. It will soon be possible to clone one hair to make as many as you need to fill in the balding areas. A dual 5-alpha-reductase inhibitor can be more potent than Propecia in inhibiting type I and II of the enzyme (Propecia only inhibits type II). There is hope that this will be FDA approved for hair loss by 2003.

Finally, says Friedman, the human genome is a major focus in treating hair loss. Now that its genes have been discovered, the question arises of what they can be used for. "It reminds me of machinists developing a hammer with no nails," he says. "It will be years before we figure out how to do something with it." Friedman says the next big solution will be cloning, which includes tissue cloning and follicle cloning. What's involved: A tiny biopsy of skin, no more than 3 millimeters in diameter and 4 millimeters deep is taken, placed into a bottle, sent to the lab for a culture, and it will be sent back with 2,000 follicles. So instead of taking the hair out of the head, it can be grown on its own. However, while this process is already being tested, the latest study says the hairs will grow but not for long before they die.

Serious Scams

Many women who suffer from hair loss are vulnerable to persuasive advertising and will try anything to get their hair back. But you can't always leap before you learn more about what you're getting into. "Most of the treatments being offered out there are a scam," says Bergfeld. "Look at what's FDA-approved or go to a physician with a national and international name in treating hair loss. Websites are helpful in identifying those doctors."

Before checking out any of the thousands of "bogus" hair care clinics around, Kingsley advises consulting with a registered qualified member of the Institute of Trichologists, preferably one that's independent of any commercial company. "Do not respond to large advertisements that promise you 'expert' or 'professional' advice and avoid those that offer 'free consultations,'" he says. "This is often used as a ploy to frighten you into signing for an expensive course of treatment." Still, those late-night infomercials can be pretty tempting. "There are a lot of commercials on television for bogus products that are coming out," says Friedman. "Many of the companies that promote products for hair loss would say they offer a money-back guarantee on any unused portion. But when a customer calls up to complain that it isn't working, they are often told that they only used the product for, say, two months and that they need to use it for three. So by the time they use it for another month, there won't be any unused portion left. Years ago, these companies were warned against this by the FDA. The bottom line is that if a product really works, it should be FDA approved."

Although there now appear to be a number of "miracle medications" and we continue to discover new scientific breakthroughs, some women simply aren't comfortable with taking pharmaceutical treatments for the rest of their lives. The good news is that there are a variety of other hair loss options, including natural and nutritional remedies.

Chapter 13

Natural and Nutritional Treatments

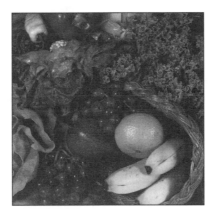

If you knew then that taking your vitamins could essentially help you hold on to your hair for a longer period of time, you just may have listened to your mom while growing up. But don't panic, there's still time to take action. When treating hair loss, if all other therapies have failed, try herbal and homeopathic remedies.

Au Natural

"There are vitamins, herbs, and supplements, like vitamin E, gingko biloba, and certain antioxidants that may or may not help with male pattern baldness, but there are no satisfactory clinical studies to substantiate any claim," says Shelly Friedman. "But although there's no proof that vitamin E, gingko biloba, and grapeseed extract actually cause hair growth, there is no downside in taking these supplements as long as you take them in the suggested daily quantities that are recommended by the manufacturer. They can be used in addition to any of the above therapies." Bergfeld shares a similar philosophy. "There are many herbals with anti-androgen activity, which may be theoretically helpful, but there is no science applied to them," she explains. "Most were produced to compete with minoxidil. For example, vitamins such as vitamin B-complex and zinc appear to be nutrients and act as blockades for the conversion of testosterone to dihydrotestosterone."

Women who are first embarking on supplemental programs should start slowly, recommends Oz Garcia, a nutritional consultant. "The dosages can be increased after a couple of weeks when you see how your body is reacting," he says. Some antioxidants he recommends include a high quality vitamin E (about 200 i.u. per day) to reduce inflammation, alpha lipoic acid (about 25 mg per day) to protect cell membranes and make other antioxidants work harder, vitamin C, ascorbic acid (about 500 mg of ester C to start). He also recommends that postmenopausal women take a high-quality antioxidant formula, like the Life Extension mix, once a day to start off their supplemental program. "Women are concerned when their

Top Ten Healthy Hair Foods

1. Salmon, cold-water fish, sardines

2. Eggs

3. Lentils

4. Wheat bran and germ

5. Kale, spinach, watercress

6. Unpolished rice

7. Cantaloupe

8. Blueberries

9. Citrus fruits

10. Seaweed

hair starts thinning or loses luster," explains chiropractor and nutritionist Mitch Peritz. "It's important to consider what you're doing with your diet, add substances that have antioxidant, anti-inflammatory, and glycating effects as well as alter your diet and add supplements that strengthen the hair."

Peritz discusses a range of supplements that are helpful in fighting hair loss, including biotin (1,000 micrograms per day), pantothenic acid (500 mg per day), vitamin B5, MSM sulfur (2,000 mg per day), and silica (500 mg per day), which comes in tablet or liquid form and strengthens hair in other ways. Biotin, which can be taken orally or injected, and dexpanthenol strengthen hair; sulfur-based amino acids, such as MSM cysteine, which comes in tablet or liquid form, are great for strengthening skin, nails, and hair. In fact, it was originally found by veterinarians who added it to the feed of horses and dogs and watched their hair and pelts get thicker. While you may be used to popping a pill or two to start your day, keep in mind that some of these supplements and nutrients come in an injectable form and can be taken via the recently popularized practice of mesotherapy. According to Lionel Bissoon, a mesotherapist based in New York City and West Palm Beach, Florida, biotin is known to be used to treat hair loss in shampoos and now can be acquired through mesotherapy. He says, "Michael Pistor, M.D., the founder of mesotherapy,

Top 12 Snacks for Super Hair

1. Almonds
2. Walnuts
3. Sunflower seeds
4. Figs
5. Apricots
6. Bananas
7. Raspberries or strawberries
8. Oranges
9. Raisins
10. Prunes
11. Skim milk, soy latte decaf, or 4 oz frozen or regular low-fat yogurt
12. Small box whole-grain cereral or whole-grain snack bar

recommends multiple injections of biotin and dexapanthenol into the scalp to give the hair and scalp the essential nutrients required for the metabolism of molecules. Some people add zinc to help build the immune system simultaneously."

Herbal Treatment List

Herbs, botanicals, and nutrients have been proven very effective for use alone or in conjunction with pharmaceutical drugs and hair transplantation surgeries. Check with your doctor, then try these options:

Saw Palmetto (*Serenosa repens*): Extract of the berries of the saw palmetto shrub slows hair loss and encourages hair regrowth. Instead of inhibiting 5-alpha-reductase, it prevents DHT from binding to the receptor sites at the prostate and hair follicles. There are no side effects, except for decreased sexual function in men, as seen with Propecia. Use saw palmetto capsules made from the berry extract that are labeled concentrated and purified with 85–95 percent fatty acids and sterols. Take one 160 mg pill in the morning and one at night.

Green Tea (*Camellia sinensis*): Green tea contains catechins, which inhibit 5-alpha-reductase and prevent the production of DHT. Green tea is also rich in antioxidants, which make it effective in treating male pattern baldness. Made from the unfermented leaves of the tea plant, it can be taken as a drink or in capsule form and has no side effects.

Pygeum (*Pygeum africanum*): From the African evergreen, pygeum inhibits 5-alpha-reductase to improve male pattern baldness. Make sure the label lists a beta sterol count of 13 percent; take 60–500 mg per day in pill or capsule form.

Stinging Nettle (*Urtica dioica*): Long used to improve the health of skin and hair, stinging nettle enhances the effects of pygeum. Take 50–100 mg per day in pill or capsule form.

Zinc: Mineral zinc inhibits the activity of 5-alpha-reductase as well as the ability of testosterone and DHT to bind to your cell's receptors, protecting the follicles from DHT and allowing for increased excretion of these hormones. The bottom line: It helps prevent and treat male pattern baldness. For optimal absorption, take 60 mg per day of zinc picolinate for six months in pill or capsule form.

That's Life

The way you live your life definitely affects the rate at which you lose your hair, mainly because stress can increase hair thinning and loss, so if you're less stressed, you might have a few extra years under cover. Environmental factors, such as exposure to pollution or toxic chemicals, can cause hair loss. Women who take birth control pills may be depleting the body of B vitamins. Those who drink alcohol and smoke deplete minerals from their bodies, which are imperative to maintaining an optimal hair lifespan. In addition, according to Mitch Peritz, daily scalp massage is rec-

Don't Eat the Oatmeal

Oatmeal may be one of your favorite breakfasts, but if you want to do right by your hair, besides eating it, wear it. Oatmeal soaps and scrubs are known for exfoliating dead, scaly skin cells that can accumulate on the scalp and soothing dry, itchy skin, dry hair, and dry scalp. Hydrolized oat protein is also an effective volumizer because it penetrates the hair shaft and reduces flyaway hair.

ommended to increase blood flow to the scalp, as will lying down on a slant board with your head down for 15 minutes per day.

Watch What You Eat

Food plays a role in the effectiveness of drug and herbal therapies when treating hair loss, so it's important to utilize food for its medicinal healing. In addition, excessive dieting or eating disorders can cause a nutritional deficiency, so it's necessary to follow certain dietary guidelines in order to protect and strengthen your hair. For example, a balanced nutritional program is essential, and since hair is made up of protein, it needs as much as possible to keep it strong. Sulfur-rich foods like beans, milk, dairy products, fish, and eggs are the basis of a healthy diet since cysteine, one of the building blocks of the hair shaft, is made of sulfur-rich amino acids. Vitamins, especially B-complex—which includes biotin—and vitamins A and C are important, as is flaxseed oil as a source of omega-3 fatty acids to improve circulation and feed the root. Wheat germ oil, which is rich in vitamin F, provides essential fatty acids to build hair. Most medical experts have their own idea of what works when it comes to diet. Here are some of their views on healthy diet programs that can make your hair stronger and look its best.

Top 10 Foods for Shine

1. Ground flax seed or oil
2. Walnuts
3. Sunflower seeds
4. Olive oil
5. Evening primrose oil
6. Ginger
7. Prunes
8. Seafood
9. Apples
10. Chickpeas

Oz Garcia, nutritional consultant and author of *The Healthy High-Tech Body*: "The most successful way of eating if you are interested in conserving the tissue of your skin and hair is with a wide variety of longevity nutrients and a high amount of omega-3 fats. The best sources of omega-3 fatty acids come from fish (salmon, tuna, mahi mahi, mackerel, and swordfish) because of the density of omega-3 fats they carry. Omega-3 fatty acids allow your body to produce all of the hormones that affect the quality of your skin and hair and work as potent lubricants for your scalp. Land-based sources of omega-3 fatty acids include olive oil, flax oil, canola oil, walnuts, and pecans."

❖

MYTH: Natural hair care products are better than "manufactured" products.

FACT: Organic products don't automatically mean better products. Organic products contain chemicals. Using something labeled organic or natural doesn't mean allergic reactions or other problems are eliminated.

❖

Garcia recommends a diet that is extremely high in a wide variety of nutrient-packed fresh, raw, and cooked vegetables, which promote longevity. Broccoli, cabbage, tomatoes, brussel sprouts, string beans, mushrooms, watercress, kale, and bok choy are beneficial on a daily basis. "Low-impact, low-glycemic carbs like rices, yams, and squashes are better for you," he says. "Be careful with high-glycemic and inflammatory carbs: pasta, bread, muffins, bagels, cookies, crackers, and cakes. They are all pro-inflammatory and tend to accelerate hair loss."

It's also important to protect against free radicals, which can damage skin and hair through oxidation, says Garcia. "Anything you consume can produce inflammatory damage caused by a retention of fluids, so that tissue may rupture and burst. It's necessary to try to control the damage of sugar in the body through glycation. Sugar molecules blend with our own tissue and cause hair follicles to age prematurely and fall out. We need to control oxidation, inflammation, and glycation through diet and supplementation."

Mitch Peritz, chiropractor and nutritionist: "Diet and nutrition is very important to maintain hair integrity. Eliminating refined foods and hydrogenated oils from the diet will help to decrease the chance of hair loss. It is important to consume a balanced diet of complex carbohydrates, protein, vegetables, and fruit to optimize the availability of nutrients, which are imperative to hair homeostasis. Essential fatty acids, including omega-3, -6, -7 and -9 should be supplemented as well. These fatty acids play a role in preventing depression and hair loss. Vegan diets are often deficient in vitamin B12 and zinc. Other things, such as B vitamins, specifically biotin (B6), folic acid (B12), and vitamin C, and minerals, including zinc, chromium, and vanadyl sulfate all play a role in stress and depression, which contribute to hair loss. High quality omega-3 fatty acids like flavored cod liver oil (try a teaspoon a day of the orange or cherry flavor from Twin Labs) will add luster. Try it for ninety days and you'll really notice a change in the quality of your hair. As far as maintaining the proper protein/carb balance, try the formula promoted by the Zone diet, which consists of 40 percent carbs, taken primarily from veggies, fruits, and low-glycemic starches, 30 percent protein, and 30 percent fat."

Did You Take Your Multivitamin Today?

"There's a cross-section of nutrients in a multivitamin that you need to maintain healthy tissues and organs throughout the body, including hair," says Jerry Hickey, nutritional pharmacist, president of Hickey Chemists and chairman of the Society of Natural Pharmacists. "Hair just won't look healthy, shiny, and lustrous unless you get the proper dose." Hickey explains that if you lack certain vitamins and nutrients, hair can become brittle or break easily, or you may experience certain scalp problems. A lack of biotin, for example, can cause yellow scales to develop on the scalp or acne to appear near the hairline. Hickey says there are other ingredients in a multivitamin that help maintain levels of antioxidants in the hair follicles—such as vitamin C, vitamin E, selenium, and carotenoids. Without them, follicles may become brittle and easily damaged. "What most people don't realize is that we need our entire system working together to maintain health," says Hickey, who recommends women take a comprehensive multivitamin every day.

make your own

An Appetite for Shine: Who says you can't eat your beans and wear them too? To increase shine and add volume, try Philip B.'s Vegetarian Refried Bean Hair Masque. He says beans make a great base for this masque because they bond to the hair. His recipe provides essential moisture to dry, damaged hair because of its high fat content.

Botanical Formula: 1 cup refried vegetarian beans, 1 avocado peeled and pitted, 8 cooked Brussels sprouts fresh or frozen, 1 cup coconut milk, 2 tablespoons chopped cooked sweet potatoes fresh or frozen, 2 tablespoons macadamia nut oil, 2 tablespoons olive oil, and 2 tablespoons canola oil. In a blender, mix all ingredients on medium-low speed until completely smooth, about 45 seconds. Apply the masque by massaging through the hair and cover with a plastic shower cap. Leave on for 10- 20 minutes then remove cap and rinse hair thoroughly with warm water, scrubbing if necessary, until mixture is completely gone. Follow with a light hair conditioner for a minute or two. Makes 2 cups.

De-Stress Yourself

Hair loss is one example of metabolic dysfunction, so it's important to maintain homeostasis or it is less likely the body will perform reparative or maintenance functions, such as heal a wound or grow hair. If you are experiencing stress, chances are you will disturb your homeostasis, or body chemistry.

Circulation is also key, according to McComb. "If we don't get nutrition to our hair follicles, they will go into a dormant phase," he says. "It's important to nourish the follicles and get blood flowing to them, since that's how they get their nutrients. Hormones affect hair follicle growth and help clean out heavy metals and improve circulation throughout the body." McComb adds that calcium and phosphorous need to be balanced in the body, and if there is an excess of toxic calcium, it can be deposited in unhealthy places, changing the balance, so this too should be avoided.

Top 10 Hair Nightmares

1. An overindulgence in carbohydrates: dry cereals, cake, soda, sugar

2. Excessive sun

3. Nylon brushes; use natural bristle

4. Drugs (to counteract the effects of antibiotics, have a cup or more of yogurt a day to help with proper absorption and digestion)

5. Allergies and infection

6. Chemicals in the form of rinses, tints, and bleaches

7. Lack of a regular scalp massage

8. Chlorine

9. Salt water

10. Bubblegum

Thyroid Troubles

"Hypothyroidism, which involves a low level of thyroid hormone, is common with women and hair loss," explains Ridha Arem, an M.D. in private practice in Houston, Texas. "The thyroid hormone affects every aspect of your metabolism, and an iron deficiency, or anemia, can directly produce hair loss." Arem explains that a decrease in iron results in a decrease in the number of red blood cells, which means that not enough oxygen is being carried to the tissues, so nutritionally hair isn't getting adequate oxidization.

The good news is that if your doctor treats the thyroid problem, your hair health will improve. "Hypo- and hyperthyroidism are both very common in women," says Valerie Peck, clinical associate professor of medicine in the department of endocrinology at New York University Medical Center. "However, the situation will improve after the thyroid has been undergoing treatment for a few months."

Fit Follicles

Stress can increase the rate of hair loss, especially when it builds up. But working out, according to Peritz, an ideal form of physical and mental release, can alleviate this stress and prevent hair loss from happening so quickly. "Stress hormones like cortisol can kill hair follicles," says Garcia. "It's important for women to work at being fit because it's a great way to regulate stress hormones. The combination of aerobic conditioning and a serious upper-body workout gives you a really good, comprehensive, well-rounded exercise program. Exercise also improves circulation, which brings blood from the capillaries to the hair follicles."

Aging Agents

"As we grow older, our life span lessens and our hair falls out faster," says Adrienne Denese, M.D., Ph.D., a specialist in antiaging medicine in private practice in Manhattan. "As the ability of the body to repair itself starts to decline, the hair follicles give up, deteriorate, and die." Denese explains that hair thickness can be measured by the number of hair follicles per unit area or by the diameter of each individual hair. "When you lose your hair, the number of hairs as well as the diameter of each hair decreases," she says. There are two types of hair: terminal hair and velous hair. "Terminal hair is the kind of hair we have when we are young," she says. "It's thick, coarse, resilient, and holds its shape nicely. Velous hair is that fluffy, strawlike hair that older women have. The individual hairs don't hold their shape at all and they grow thin in diameter, so they are more fragile. As we age, more and more hair turns velous until, eventually, all of our hair is velous. For this reason, most older women keep their hair short since it looks healthier."

Denese explains that as we age, our bodies don't make enough protein for our hair to repair itself properly and it begins to deteriorate. In addition, our growth hormone levels decrease as we age and because of this our hair grows progressively drier. Diet has a minimal effect as well. "When you're young, make sure you have all the essential fatty acids to make your hair a bit more shiny," says Denese. "An older person can take all the fatty acids they want but they'll be of minimal help since years of sunlight dries out and damages hair."

As you can see, living a healthy life with a balanced diet, physical exercise, and minimal stress can even have a positive effect on your hair! And taking vitamins and herbal remedies appear beneficial as well. But, if none of the methods you've tried have succeeded, don't despair—hair transplants and grafts can create the natural appearance you desire.

Strike a Pose

Nutrition and exercise are important for keeping fit and healthy, and that includes keeping hair healthy. "The growth of our hair is related to the thyroid, and when people experience trauma, the thyroid shuts down and our hair can turn gray or fall out," explains Deansin Goodson Parker, Ph.D., owner of the Goodson Parker Wellness Center and coauthor of *Yoga Baby*. "In yoga, there are movements and poses you can do to stimulate the thyroid gland, which will in turn determine the shape of your hair and skin and the nature of the endocrine system. When the thyroid gland is functioning properly, new hair growth is stimulated." Not all medical experts agree with this theory, but gentle exercise and stretching is great for the circulation and for your fitness level—and that's good for your hair. Here are two easy movements that can help:

The Cobra: Lie on the floor on your stomach with your legs outstretched and your hands at your sides. Push your pubic bone into the floor and lift from the chest to bring your torso off the floor, hold for a few seconds and release.

The Shoulder Stand: Lie on your back with your hands supporting your lower back and then stretch your legs toward the ceiling. Maintain this hold for a minute with a coordinated breath. Return from the position slowly and carefully.

Head Cases

Imagine that every time you took a shower, brushed your hair, or pulled on a turtleneck, you found clumps of hair in your hand, in your towel, on your bathroom floor. The women you're about to meet did. After searching for a cure, they each found a solution that worked for them. Here's how some women cured their hair loss blues.

✦

I've always had thin, fine hair. I had a lot of it so it never seemed like it was as fine as it was. I always thought we had bad hair in my family because thinning, graying hair is hereditary. I didn't color my hair until my late thirties. I started coloring it with gentle, over-the-counter hair color products and my hair started falling out, really badly, everywhere. My cleaning lady couldn't believe it; she kept asking me whose hair she was finding all over the house. For the most part, it was all because of the coloring process. I was starting to feel very down about the way my hair looked. I was determined to not have my mother's problem hair. I wanted to do something before it got too late. I knew I needed a hairstyle that didn't require curl because I can't perm my hair.

I heard about Lynn Glaze at Sheer Reflections. She is a master stylist and a specialist in hair color. I also had a friend who went to her for her hair color and really liked her, so I decided to pay her a visit. She started using a Paul Mitchell hair color beeswax, typically for fine hair, on my hair, and in no time, I could see the drastic difference—my hair looked shinier and healthier. My hair was also really dry, so I began using Paul Mitchell shampoos, hair moisture mist, and heat sealer. I was a good student and did exactly what she told me to do religiously.

After about a year, I started using Rogaine and my hair quit falling out. It's not as long as I'd like it to be, but I still have a hard time getting it to grow. However, I don't have as many really aggressive split ends as I used to have, so my hair is in much better shape all the way around, and I'm not losing it the way I had been.

Lynn also advised me on different tools and products that really made a difference. I still use the heat sealer product. She also said I didn't need to use a round brush on my hair if I was using a curling iron.

My advice to other women who are suffering from hair loss is that if you have problem hair, which I do, you have to have a professional treat it. I went to a lot of people before I met Lynn. Now I feel better about my hair. I will never like the fact that I need to wash it every day, but I have minimal hair loss at this point. And I'll always know what I'm doing as far as taking care of my hair.—Vickie, 43, Alexandria, Louisiana

✦

I first went to Lynn Glaze for a styling problem. I had given myself a bad home perm and everywhere I went, professionals told me I just had to grow it out and that they couldn't fix it. A friend told me about Lynn, so I made an appointment. Lynn tested my hair and gave it a heat treatment where it was split and fried. This was four years ago, and I have been letting it grow out since. Then, about two years ago, my hair started falling out. I thought it was the usual everyday stress; after all, I work hard and have three children and I was going through a problem with one of my teenagers. I noticed that everywhere I looked—in my towels after a shower, when I washed my clothes and dried them, there were strands of hair. I noticed it most around my temples and I noticed I had a really bad dry scalp with scabs that was so itchy that I scratched it all the time. I told Lynn it had been going on for about six months, and she said the dry scalp was causing my hair to fall out. She felt it probably wasn't hormonal but rather a genetic thing. I don't have anyone in my family who has suffered this. I kept thinking I couldn't imagine wearing wigs and hats all the time.

But Lynn knew just what to do. She put me on a hydrating botanical shampoo and creme rinse and my scalp felt wonderful. It wasn't itchy or scaly or scabbed over and I found I wasn't scratching it. The tub didn't look as bad as it used to. Before using the products, I was able to collect as much hair throughout the day to make a small six-inch square pillow. Not anymore. In addition, soon I began to notice little bitsy hair sprouts growing in and I knew my hair was growing back. I even get my hair highlighted and the highlights lift my fine thin hair and give it body.

If I go away for the weekend and use the shampoo in the hotel bathroom, my scalp starts itching again. My advice to others: If you can't talk openly to your hairdresser about your hair, or if he/she can't talk to you about it, you need to go somewhere else.—Marcia, 37, Louisiana

✦

I was diagnosed with ovarian cancer and I was completely in denial. I knew I had to have chemotherapy and that my hair would fall out, but I still couldn't believe it was happening. Everything seemed so surreal. I had heard that most chemo patients experience thinning.

When I first started to notice it, I signed up for a free consultation with Joelle, a stylist at the Avon Salon in New York City who runs a special program for cancer patients to help them deal with losing their hair. I have fine hair but a lot of it, and I haven't worn it short since I was a teenager. Joelle's assessment was for me to cut my hair in stages, and keep going shorter to get me used to having no hair. For the first cut, she didn't drastically cut it all off, she just took it to the next level.

When I started, it was about three inches below my shoulders and she cut it to above my shoulders. Then two weeks later, I was in the shower and my hair just started coming out in clumps. I figured I would make an appointment to see her the next week and get the next cut, but all of my hair came out within the next two days. I literally had to run to the wig shop to buy a wig.

I found one that was bilevel, and slightly above shoulder length. It was made of a mix of synthetic and natural hair so it's easier to maintain and is lighter. Wearing a wig was difficult for me at first, especially since I don't like to wear hats. I'll wear a baseball cap when I'm working out or a ski cap when I'm skiing, but any other time, I get a headache from them.

I have to tape it down to keep it in place. When I first wore it, I kept thinking I'd be walking down 57th Street on a windy day saying, "Whoops! There goes my hair." Another fear was that everyone would know I was wearing one. One day my boss said, "I love your hair!" and I said "Do you want to borrow it?" It was funny. No one could tell it was a wig. Another funny thing is that I used to spend $200 a month getting my hair done, half an hour in the morning getting it conditioned and blow-dried, but now I just have to cut a piece of tape and make sure I put it on correctly, then stick the wig on my head.

I'm more comfortable with it, but it still feels like a wig. Sometimes it feels a little warm, but it's not too bad and some days I can feel it around the crown. Sometimes I just can't wait to go home at the end of the day and rip it off my head and put on a bandanna. And if I'm out with friends and I stay out too late at night, I still have to have time to wash my wig with ample time for it to dry. I can't use a blow dryer on it, so I have to do it the night before.

Last week, I was out and two men tried to pick me up and I was relieved that now my hair always looks great. One was bald so I thought, "That's appropriate," and the other guy thought I was hot. At least the wig was doing some good!—Mary, 38, New York City

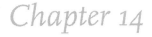

Chapter 14

Surgical Treatments

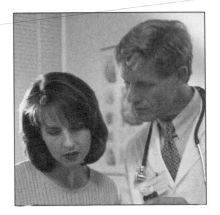

If you've tried shampoos, medicines, and the latest style wig and still don't feel comfortable with your lack of or thinning hair, consider these surgical procedures designed to give you a fuller head of follicles. Some have serious side effects or unruly results, so consult a physician and find the one that's right for you before going under the knife.

Looking to Relocate: Hair Transplants

Hair transplants consist of removing hair plugs of varying sizes from areas where the hair is continuing to grow (the donor area) and placing them in areas where hair has been lost (the recipient area). Donor areas are usually found in the back of the scalp, which rarely goes bald. The plugs are spaced slightly apart to enable the surrounding tissue to assist in feeding the transplanted sections. It offers a tufted appearance, but follow-up micrografts or minigrafts can fill them in with one, two, or three hairs to help create a more natural appearance. The donor hair in back and on the lower sides is rarely if ever lost, and the follicles, which produce that hair, will do so throughout your lifetime. When those follicles are moved in transplantation to an area of thinning hair or baldness, they will keep the characteristics of their original location and continue to produce hair. This concept is called donor dominance.

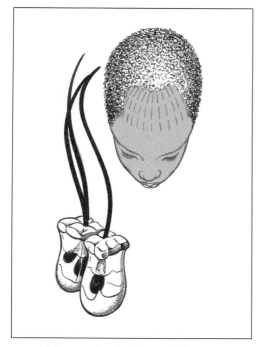

Hair transplanting is one of the most natural-looking hair regrowth procedures on the market.

It's important to remember that since the recipient area can't grow hair, the hairs surrounding the transplanted hair will continue to thin, leaving patches of transplanted hair. So save some recipient areas for touch-up surgeries later on. Also remember that this procedure can cause minor scarring in the donor areas and carries a modest risk for skin infection. The procedure usually requires multiple transplantation sessions and may be expensive.

The good news: "Hair follicles that aren't sensitive to dihydrotestosterone can be moved to another area, and they will maintain the color, characteristics, and genetic longevity of healthy hair," says Dr. Friedman. "You live to your 80s and it will still be growing." According to Friedman, hair transplants can be taken from an identical twin but not from a general family member, because it is essential to obtain the right tissue type. "When donating organs, even with the right tissue type, the recipient would still have to be on antirejection antibodies to prevent her own body from rejecting the donor organ. These drugs open up the possibility of infection, something that just wouldn't be done for a cosmetic procedure. Maybe someday there will be drugs that are tissue specific and can be targeted to only the hair follicles."

The Goods on Grafting: Hair Grafts

In the old days, there were hair plugs that were so far from subtle they could be spotted a mile away. Strips of hair were cut out from the back of the head, which had to be stitched back up, leaving an ugly scar. Follicular units were removed and then replanted into the barer areas at random. Today, according to Steven Victor, a cosmetologist in private practice in New York City, grafting is one of the most natural-looking hair re-growth procedures on the market. "This procedure involves the grafting of one or two follicular units in an effort to get natural-looking hair that re-creates what nature gave us. Those are called micrografts. In a minigraft, three to five follicular units

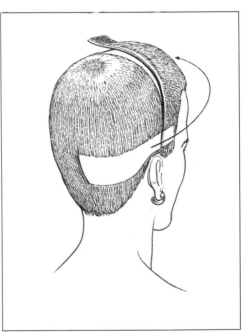

Most surgeons do not recommend the procedure called a hair flap; the results don't look natural, and the procedure itself is painful.

in the same piece of skin are transplanted. We do micrografts closer to the front and minigrafts behind. The problem is if there aren't enough hairs growing out of each pore it won't look natural because hairs will be too spread out. Most doctors tend to use micrographs about 80 percent of the time and a combination of micrografts and minigrafts in about 20 percent of their cases."

"Grafting is a great option for women who have diffused hair loss and want a particular area thickened up," says Victor. "But for every hundred guys who undergo a surgical hair procedure, there is probably one woman who does so as well. Hair loss tends to be obvious in men because of distribution on top and in the front. Women have estrogen protecting them, but in general hair loss tends to be diffused all over the scalp of a woman. Instead of bald patches, hair gets thinner all over and there is no sizable donor area."

To Flap or not to Flap: Hair Flaps

In this procedure, a sizable strip of scalp is taken from its original

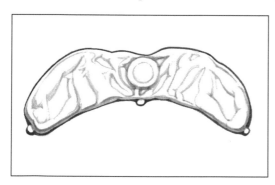

Again, most surgeons do not recommend having a soft tissue expansion done. Unsightly scars can result.

home base and transposed to an area that is balding to produce normal density hair in that area. It is a serious procedure that involves anesthesia. Only a small percentage of patients (about 15 to 20 percent, some female) are good candidates because their hair loss is restricted to a small frontal area. Hair styling and treatment tricks can be used to minimize the appearance of hair that grows backward, or the flap can be designed so that there's more forward-growing hair. Flaps are done over a week in different stages, to allow time for the "lump" or "dog-ear" in the area where the flap has been turned to grow into the scalp. The final stage is the surgical correction of the dog-ear to return the flap in the hairline to its normal appearance.

The flap depends on the artery that it is feeding off is for survival. Over two to four weeks after it is sewn into its new home, it develops blood supply from this new location and is divided from its original base by cutting off the artery.

The benefits of flaps are that they create a beautiful anterior hairline with excellent hair density. The downside is that not everyone is a candidate since they may not have the right distribution of hair loss. It is essential to do the procedure on patients whose primary area of baldness is near the front. In addition, since it takes a number of stages, you can't just get it over with. Expect and plan for recovery time!

Expand Your Horizons: Soft Tissue Expanders

Years ago, if an area was too large to be transplanted, the hair-bearing area of the scalp was stretched to expand the area that will be covered by hair. This was done with the insertion of a silicone balloon into a pocket between the scalp and the skull (unsightly scars are likely to result). Over a period of weeks, the balloon is blown up. In response to enlarging the balloon, the hair-bearing tissue of the scalp (not the number of hair-bearing follicles) expands, increasing the area of donation by mini- and micrografting or flap transfer. This is a great benefit to flap surgery. Once hair is transposed, closure is easier because there is more scalp tissue to work with.

Faux Follicles: Implanting Artificial Fibers

Implanting artificial fibers into the scalp is another option for creating new "hair." How it works: Synthetic fibers are implanted in small bundles directly into your scalp. The procedure can cause the scalp's natural oils to build up at the base, resulting in inflammation and infection, which can destroy the scalp. In addition, the fibers are brittle and can frizz or break easily. Styling and blow-drying can also permanently damage them. The bottom line, as most experts will agree, is that it doesn't look or feel like real hair. Another important issue: It can get inflamed or infected.

Do the Weave: Hair Weaving

Hair weaving, hairpieces, or change of hairstyle may disguise the hair loss and improve the cosmetic appearance. This is often the least expensive and safest method of treating female pattern baldness. Hair weaving involves weaving together a fine net with hair attached and your natural hair. Hair is woven as close to the scalp as possible. Scalp friction can cause irritation and infection, and the procedure needs to be repeated about every other month since the net is raised farther away from the scalp as the hair grows. Also, weaves often pull on your hair underneath the hairpiece, causing traction alopecia, or localized hair loss. Hair weaving should be done carefully by an expert to ensure that tension placed on hair is minimal or it can cause severe hair loss.

MYTH: Standing on one's head or getting a head massage will increase circulation and stimulate hair growth.

FACT: Increasing circulation in the scalp certainly can't hurt, but it will not stimulate hair growth.

Integration Nation: Hair Integration

Hair integration is another option. Human hair is integrated with your own hair through a network of small, gold cylinders that attach the new hair to your hair. Using the cylinders allows more breathing room for your hair and looks natural but can be costly to maintain.

Essential Cutback: Scalp Reductions

If the bald area is too large to cover with the limited amount of hair available on the donor site, the surface area of the bald section must be reduced. Now fairly common, a two-inch patch of scalp is removed, bringing the two hair-bearing pieces of scalp at the sides closer together. Once the skin is healed, hair can be transplanted onto the remaining area. Some resulting problems can include a hideous scar where the edges of the sections meet, accelerated hair loss, scalp thinning, an unnatural direction of hair growth, infection, hemorrhaging, pain and swelling from sutures, and loosened skin when the stitches relax.

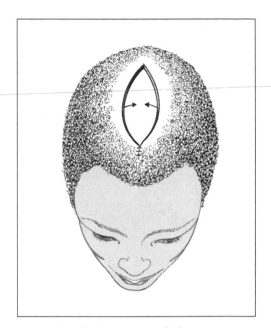

Scalp reduction is now a fairly common procedure, but its side effects may give pause to most of us.

Tissue expansion can help here as well. One of the problems with scalp reduction is that when the scars get wide, they're thick and unattractive. If the hair-bearing tissue is expanded before scalp reduction, the reduction is easier and scars are less likely to widen or become cosmetically unacceptable. In addition, a new type of expander that looks like a stretchy rubber sheet is placed under the scalp, stretched from side to side, and attached on both ends. It pulls the side up toward the top of the scalp and contracts the inside of the scalp, minimizing ugly scars that can result from scalp reduction.

A Stitch in Time: Suturing the Scalp

Simply stated, suturing involves stitching fake hair to the scalp. Suturing of hairpieces to the scalp is not recommended, as it can result in scars, infections, and abscess of the scalp or brain. A thin layer of scar tissue replaces the skin, and these scars may cause blockage of the blood supply to the central portion of the scalp. Since the sutures aren't ever removed and don't dissolve, they tend to cut through the skin and have to be replaced. Combing your hair may also pull at the sutures and loosen them. Eventually, there's a good chance your scalp may reject the sutured hair. Finally, the area of natural hair around the sutured hair can be permanently destroyed.

All of these procedures require considered thought before undertaking them. They are all serious operations and, given some of the dangerous side effects of some of these surgical treatments, it's absolutely essential to choose a qualified specialist.

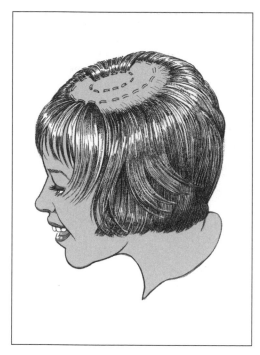

Suturing is another iffy procedure and can cause infection, scarring, and worse.

Chapter 15

Is There a Doctor in the House?

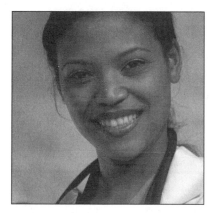

So you're thinking of having hair surgery, but trying to find a specialist can leave you pulling (the rest of) your hair out. There's no need to panic; there are hundreds of physicians around who can get the job done effectively, safely, and with minimal discomfort, leaving you looking and feeling great.

"Hair transplant surgery can be performed by many types of doctors across the board from family medical practitioners, general plastic surgeons, heart surgeons, vascular surgeons, facial plastic surgeons, dermatologists, and others," explains Mark Glasgold, M.D., a facial and plastic surgeon, based in Highland Park, New Jersey, and in Manhattan. "Some of them may have naturally expanded into these areas, others may have decided they didn't like their original specialty and pursued a specialty in hair transplant surgery. There are no qualifications in basic training that makes one person better than another. In fact, one of best transplant surgeons in the country used to be a psychiatrist."

"Choosing the right specialist is extremely important," says Robert Guida, M.D., director of facial and plastic surgery at New York Hospital Cornell Medical Center. "A doctor can be board certified as an emergency medical physician or a podiatrist, but that doesn't mean he/she can do hair transplants. There are even OB/GYNs who do liposuction as well as hair transplants. It's very important to find someone who has done a good number of hair surgeries and keeps up to date on the latest techniques." Dr. Guida adds that you shouldn't feel restricted to looking for a physician in your own area. "If you live in a big city, you'll find a handful of very good hair surgeons, but if you live in a rural area, you may have limited options and it might be worth traveling a bit to find someone more qualified. For example, if you live in central Illinois, it might be worth traveling to Chicago to have your surgery done. It will be worth the trip. "

Do You Really Need to Go Under the Knife?

Just because you arrange a consultation with a hair surgeon doesn't mean you are going to need surgery. The right surgeon will examine you and try to treat your hair loss with medications first. "The advantage to coming in early," says Tom Rosanelli, M.D., chairman of the American Society of Hair Restoration Surgery, a subgroup of the American Academy of Cosmetic Surgery, "is that there are several drugs currently available on the market to prevent hair loss making it possible to stop hair loss prior to surgery. This can allow a patient to go several more years before undergoing a surgical procedure."

If you have experienced a minimal amount of hair loss or thinning but are okay with that and just don't want to experience further hair loss, you can be treated medically for the rest of your life. The doctor should be able to listen to a patient's expectations and desires and treat him/her accordingly.

Getting Credit: Find a Doctor with a Degree that Counts

"There are surgeons from different specialties that perform hair replacement surgery," says Dr. Rosanelli, "but the only board that can specifically certify a doctor in hair replacement surgery is the American Board of Hair Restoration Surgery. If a physician is not a member of this board, it's important to find out what experience he/she has in hair restoration." There are two organizations that teach procedures and offer conferences in hair restoration surgery: The International Society of Hair Restoration Surgery and the American Society of Hair Restoration Surgery. Says Dr. Rosanelli, "If a doctor isn't certified by the American Board of Hair Restoration Surgery or isn't a member of either of these organizations, it's not the best sign. On the other hand, just because a doctor is a member of either of these societies, doesn't necessarily mean he/she's qualified."

"These organizations are legitimate bodies and the people who run them are focused on producing good results, avoiding confrontation, and taking good care of patients," explains Dr. Mark Glasgold, M.D. "There are also a number of great websites available that list surgeons in your area. Keep in mind, however, that a lot of people are able to travel successfully before and after hair transplant surgery since there is little post-op care. The procedure is done and then you leave." Apparently, there is no certification for hair surgery within the certification for dermatology or plastic surgery. So while these practitioners may have experience practicing hair restoration surgery, they won't be specifically certified for it.

Dr. Rosanelli advises potential hair surgery candidates to find out the number of years a physician has been doing surgery, look at before-and-after photos of previous patients and, if possible, speak to a former patient about his/her experience with the doctor and the procedure. "The amount of experience a doctor has is critical in this particular field, no matter how much experience he/she has as a surgeon. If a doctor hasn't practiced hair surgery, a number of things can go wrong."

According to Dr. Rosanelli, one or two hair surgeries a year aren't enough to give a surgeon enough experience. In fact, doctors who specialize in hair surgery procedures often do somewhere between twenty to forty cases a year. "A surgeon should be doing five cases a month to stay current. The American Board of Hair Restoration Surgery requires fifty cases a year to qualify to take the board."

"I think you have to use your common sense and get several consults before you decide to do the procedure," says Thomas Romo III, M.D., F.A.C.S., director of facial, plastic, and reconstructive surgery at Lenox Hill Hospital and Manhattan Eye, Ear and Throat in New York City. "It's also important for a person to know what's going on with new technology. You don't want to go to the first person who's doing a new procedure, but you don't want to go to the last person, either."

Do's and Don'ts of Choosing a Specialist

There are so many questions to ask, so much research to be done. Thus before you sign on the dotted line, check out this list of do's and don'ts for choosing a hair surgeon.

Do

- Ask around for a referral. "The best way to find a doctor is by personal recommendation or word of mouth," says Dr. Guida. "Ask around among family, friends, and colleagues and see which physicians' names routinely come up."

- Ask to see pictures of the doctor's patients before and after their surgeries. If the procedure was done correctly, you won't be able to tell they had anything done at all. "Look at the results critically without seeing a smiling face with a full head of hair," says Dr. Glasgold. "Detailed pictures of frontal hairlines will tell all. Fine dark hair on light skin is the most difficult transplant. If someone has trouble creating a frontal hairline it will show. Also, keep in mind that you're evaluating that person's best work. And if you're not impressed by their best work, you won't be impressed by their average work."

- Ask for contact information to ensure that these are actually patients of this particular doctor; ask for the contact information to confirm these previous patients' experiences and their results. Meet with them and look at their hair. After all, seeing is believing.

Don't

- Don't pursue a doctor who claims he/she doesn't have pictures of patients. "My camera's broken" falls into the same category as "The dog ate my homework."

- Don't waste time with a doctor who shows you mass-produced brochures featuring patients that aren't their own. If you've seen the same pictures at another doctor's office, you have reason to doubt them.

What's Up, Doc? Interview Your Doctor

First and foremost, you need to feel comfortable with this surgeon. "Make sure you meet the surgeon and feel comfortable with him/her so that if something goes wrong, you know you can go back for help," says Dr. Glasgold. "You want to find someone who looks at you like a patient, not a customer, and cares about your medical issues." While the doctor needs to interview you to find out if you are a good candidate, you also need to interview the doctor to find out if he is qualified at what he does and if he understands your expectations. "It's important for patients to interview their physicians," says Dr. Romo. "There are a lot of doctors out there and you need to make sure they have the training in what you want them to do. I have no problem with patients asking me to tell them about the results, complications, progress of my last hundred surgeries."

"It's helpful to go to someone who specializes in hair surgery but, if not, you want to at least use someone who has performed a good number of surgeries," says Dr. Guida. "You don't want to use someone who only does this once a month or a few times a year, since they won't have as much experience as other doctors who have done it more often."

Here are some key questions to ask:

Do you have your own team of technicians? Find out how much the technicians actually do. You don't want to use someone who lets techs do all the work but, at the same time, you want to ensure there is a qualified team of assistants to help with the procedure.

Am I a good candidate for hair surgery? "Ask the doctor whether or not you are an easy transplant," suggests Dr. Glasgold. "Are there areas where it may take more than one procedure to meet your expectations? Will he do one procedure to move 15,000 hairs over the course of eight hours or will he do three two-hour sessions?"

What techniques do you use? If you look at the pictures and see big plugs that look unnatural, that's what you will get. But if the surgeon is using the right combination of mini- and micrografts or follicular transplants, the results will look extremely natural. "Follicular transplant is state-of-the-art," says Dr. Glasgold. "Not every transplant has to be done using this procedure, but a surgeon who uses it shows a sign of someone who is maintaining a current level of technique and technology and is always working to improve his skills."

What specific procedure will you use for me? It doesn't matter whether the doctor knows how to perform all of the general hair surgery procedures. Each treatment plan should be individualized for each patient, and the doctor should be able to explain what he plans to do for you. For example, will the doctor do follicular transplants all around or will he mix follicular transplants in the frontal region with some micrografts in other areas? You should also be able to look at pictures of someone with hair similar to yours to give you as much of an idea of what to expect.

How qualified are you to perform hair surgery? "When I do surgery, I like to get good results, but hair surgery is not my specialty," says Dr. Glasgold. "So while I tend to operate on more favorable patients—those with lighter or curly hair—and I have done quite a few transplants, I will send patients who require more detailed procedures to someone who is devoted to doing hair."

What other medications can I take simultaneously, or what hormones can I be on? Your doctor should be able to advise you on medications and hormones that you may take during the pre- and post-op period.

Can the doctor offer nutritional and endocrinological advice to help you deal with the procedure? The doctor should also focus on hair physiology as well as hair surgery. He/she should be able to provide nutritional counseling and should give you a complete physical analysis beforehand to check for thyroid gland problems as well as autoimmune disease. If the doctor doesn't feel comfortable discussing these issues, he/she should be able to refer you to a nutritionist or endocrinologist who can offer expert advice.

How much will this cost? "Price is based on how much hair needs to be moved," says Dr. Glasgold, "so there is a huge range of prices around the market. You can find tremendous bargains out there, so it's worth shopping around. Just keep in mind that quality isn't synonymous with price."

Get a Face Lift, Lose Your Hair: Can Other Plastic Surgeries Affect Hair Loss?

The last thing you want to do is go in for a face lift, rhinoplasty, eyelid blepharoplasty, or any other facial surgery and find that in order to do the procedure, the doctor has cut away critical masses of hair-bearing skin. Lucky for us, surgeons like Dr. Romo are sure to take this into consideration before embarking on creating your new look.

"As a surgeon, the last thing I want to do is cut out hair-bearing skin, even when doing a face lift. So I developed a way to do face lifts, eyelid blepharoplasties, and other surgical procedures by making an incision at the hair line instead of going back into the hair where extra skin can be cut away."

Dr. Romo explains that the upper part of the face, including the eyelids, brows, and forehead, ages a decade before the lower part does. "People used to come in for consults in their 50s and 60s," says Dr. Romo. "Now, they show up in their late 30s and 40s." He explains that the previous procedure for people who came in with redundant upper eyelid skin was to cut away the excess or to pull the eyebrows up toward the hairline when they begin to droop down.

The technique used involved making an incision from ear to ear across the top of the head 6 centimeters from the frontal hairline, which is called a coronal brow lift. Through this process, an incision is made in the hair-bearing skin and the skin is pulled back, then one inch of hair-bearing skin is cut out and thrown away. In an endoscopic brow/forehead lift, which Dr. Romo now performs, a small incision is made in the hairline, and the brows are pulled into place and secured via sutures into the bone. The skin then shrink-wraps down to the skull and no hair-bearing skin is removed. "This is a more conservative technique which gets the job done and helps maintain hair growth," says Dr. Romo.

Armed with this information in mind, you are set to seek out a professional who can help you look and feel your best by restoring your hair to a close-to-natural state. The bottom line: Do your homework and you'll reap the rewards.

Resources

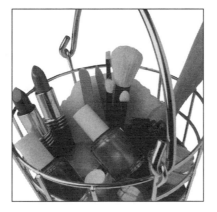

Premier Products

It takes great products to keep your hair looking its best. But if you don't want to make the trip to your local drug store, department store, or beauty salon to stock up, check out our list of contact numbers and websites where you can place your order.

Alberto Culver: Shampoos, conditioners, and hair care products,
(708) 450-3000
www.alberto.com

Aquage: Sea-inspired professional shampoos, conditioners, styling, and
finishing products,
(877) 238-1100

ARTec: A professional line of salon products developed by hairdressers for
hairdressers and a favorite of consumers,
(800) 323-6817
www.artecworldwide.com

Aveda: Botanical-based skin care, hair, and make-up and spa products,
(800) 328-0849, (800) 283-3224
www.aveda.com

Avon: A wide variety of beauty, hair, and makeup products,
(800) FOR-AVON (367-2866)
www.avon.com

Bath & Body Works: Shampoos, conditioners,
and hair care products,
(800) 395-1001
www.bathandbodyworks.com

Bioelements: The makers of Bio, a comprehensive collection
of hair care and hairstyling products for all hair types,
(800) 433-6650
www.bioelements.com

Bio Ionic: Professional hair products and tools that smooth
and straighten hair via the ionic system,
(310) 273-9001
www.bioionic.com

Black and Beautiful: Conditioning, strengthening, and treatment
products for hair,
(877) 811-9709
www.blackandbeautiful.info

Breck, a Himmel Company: The first shampoo in America, Breck offers a
complete line of hair care products,
(866) 273-2574

Bumble and Bumble: Hair cutting, styling, and treatment products,
(800) 7-BUMBLE
www.bumbleandbumble.com

Charles Worthington: Salon owner, celebrity stylist, and hair products
for men and women,
(800) 519-8121
www.cwlondon.com

Citre Shine: Shampoos, conditioners, and styling products,
(714) 556-1028
www.citreshine.com

Clairol: Shampoos, conditioners, and home hair color products,
(800) 223-5800
www.clairol.com or
www.herbalessences.com

Clinique: Skin care and makeup, plus a new line of hair care products, including shampoos, conditioners, shaping, styling, and shine products, (800) 419-4041
www.clinique.com

Conair: Hair dryers, curling irons, electric rollers, brushes, combs, and other styling tools, (800) 3-CONAIR
www.conair.com

Elizabeth Arden: A full range of beauty, hair, and makeup products and services, (800) 99-ARDEN
www.reddoorsalons.com

Eufora International: Hair-styling tools, (800) 6-Eufora
www.eufora.net

Frédéric Fekkai: Hair-cleansing and styling products, salon and spa services, (888) FFEKKAI (333-5524)
www.fredericfekkai.com

Freeman: A full range of well-priced hair and skin care products, www.freemancosmetics.com

Fudge: Hair treatment and styling products, (800) 383-4387
www.fudge.com

Galderma: The makers of Capex dandruff shampoo, (817) 961-5000
www.capexshampoo.com

Garren New York Hair Care Collection: Performance-based cleansing, conditioning, and styling products with natural plant extracts and a New York salon,
(877) 441-9255
www.garrennewyork.com

Goldwell: Professional-only haircare products,
(888) 881-0330
www.goldwellusa.com

Head and Shoulders: Antidandruff shampoo and conditioner,
(800) 723-9569
www.headandshoulders.com

Helene Curtis: Shampoos, conditioners, and home hair color products,
(800) 782-8301
www.helenecurtis.com

Hill Dermaceuticals: The makers of Derma-Smoothe/FS Scalp Oil,
(800) 344-5707
www.hillderm.com

Jean Pierre Paris: Brushes, combs, and other styling tools,
(877) JPIERRE
www.jean-pierre-creations.com

J. F. Lazartigue: French botanical hair treatment products and hair analysis,
(212) 288-2250
www.jflazartigue.com

John Frieda: Hair-styling products and salons,
(800) 521-3189
www.johnfrieda.com

Joico: Shampoos, conditioners, and styling products,
(800) 44-JOICO
www.joico.com

Kérastase: Hair treatment and styling products,
(877) 748-8357
www.kerastase.com

KMS: Hair treatment and styling products,
(800) 342-5567
www.kmshaircare.com

L'Oréal: A full range of beauty, hair, and makeup products, including
over-the- counter hair color,
(800) 631-7358; (800) 322-2036
www.lorealparis.com

Mason Pearson: High quality brushes and combs,
(516) 599-1776
www.masonpearson.com

Matrix: Shampoos, conditioners, and other hair care and styling products,
(800) 282-2822
www.matrixbeautiful.com

Neutrogena: Hair and skin care products, including shampoos, conditioners, soaps, and bath items,
(800) 421-6857
www.neutrogena.com

Nexxus: Shampoos, conditioners, styling products, and hair repair treatments,
(800) 444-6399
www.nexxus.com

Nioxin: Hair regrowth products,
(800) 628-9890
www.nioxin.com

Nizoral: Antidandruff shampoo and non-medicated conditioner,
(800) 962-5357
www.nizoral.com

OSIS: An advanced formula styling collection created by hairdressers for the hairdresser,
(800) 707-9997
www.schwarzkopf.com

Ouidad: Curly hair specialist with dedicated salon and products,
(800) 677-4247
www.ouidad.com

Pantene: Shampoos, conditioners, and other hair care and styling products,
(800) 945-7768
www.pantene.com

Paul Mitchell: Professional salons nationwide and professional scalp therapy shampoos, conditioners, and other hair care and styling products,
(800) 793-8790
www.paulmitchell.com

Philip B.: Specialty hair care products sold to selective salons and stores,
(800) 643-5556
www.philipb.com

Physique: Cleansing, shaping, and styling products,
(800) 214-8957
www.physique.com

PHYTO: Hair care and styling products,
(800) 55-PHYTO
www.phyto.com

Prive: Celebrity hair salon and makers of shampoos, conditioners, and styling products,
(866) 351-1193
www.priveproducts.com

Redken: Shampoo, conditioner, hair color, and other hair care and styling products,
(800) REDKEN-8 (733-5368)
www.redken.com

Rene Furterer: Hair care and styling products,
(800) 522-8285
www.renefurterer.com

Revlon: A full line of beauty, hair, and makeup products,
(800) 4-REVLON
www.revlon.com

Ricky's: Sells a full range of hair and beauty products,
(212) 352-8545
www.rickys-nyc.com

Rogaine: A complete line of hair regrowth products,
(800) ROGAINE (764-2463)
www.rogaine.com

Rusk: A complete line of hair care products, as well as technical assistance,
(800) 873-7875
www.rusk1.com

Sally Beauty Supply: Sells a full range of hair and beauty products
from shampoos, conditioners, and treatment products to styling tools,
(800) 275-7255
www.sallybeauty.com

Salon Selectives: Shampoos, conditioners, mousse, and other hair care
and styling products,
(866) 266-5367
www.salonselectives.com

Schwarzkopf: A leading hair color and hair care company, Schwarzkopf
is the choice of the world's most celebrated hair stylists and colorists,
(800) 707-9997
www.schwarzkopf.com

Sebastian International: The makers of several different hair care
productlines,
(800) 829-7322
www.sebastian-intl.com

St. Ives: A full range of well-priced hair and skin care products,
(818) 709-5500
www.stives.com

Suave: A full range of well-priced hair and skin care products,
(800) 782-8301
www.suave.com

Thicker Fuller Hair: Hair-thickening shampoos, conditioners,
and leave-in products,
(714) 556-1028 ext. 232
www.thickerfuller.com

Vidal Sassoon: Professional hair care products and salons nationwide,
(800) 262-1637
www.vidalsassoon.com

White Rain Co.: A full range of well-priced hair care products including
White Rain and Dippity Do,
(800) 872-7202 or (800) 575-7960
www.whiterain.com or
www.whiteraincompany.com

Perfect Accessories

You can give your hair a new twist with the right accessories. Look
for these designer names to check out the latest looks:

Brad Johns Colorsave Haircare Products: Sold at Avon Salon and Spa,
Trump Tower, 725 Fifth Avenue at 56th Street, New York, NY; (212) 755-AVON

Colette Malouf: For information on where to buy accessories contact Malouf, Colette Inc., 594 Broadway, Suite 1216, New York, NY 10012; (212) 941-9588

Dolce & Gabbana: Sold at Dolce & Gabbana boutiques; go to www.dolcegabbana.it for store locations

Emanuel Ungaro: Go to www.emanuelungaro.com for store locations

Erickson Beamon: Sold at Barneys New York; go to www.barneys.com for store locations

Eve Reid: Sold at Sephora.com; go to www.sephora.com for store locations

Marc by Marc Jacobs: Sold at Marc Jacobs boutiques; go to www.marcjacobs.com for store locations and to www.eluxury.com

Shaneed Huxham: Sold at CO Bigelow Chemist, 414 6th Avenue, between 8th and 9th Street; for further store information about where Shaneed Huxham hair accessories are sold, call (212) 947-4255

Contributing Experts

From how to take care of it when you have it to how to deal with losing it, these experts were gracious enough to devote their time to *The Hair Bible* to help you understand the hair care process:

Aleta St. James: New York City–based emotional healer; telephone, (865) 546-0000; fax, (865) 673-4680; e-mail, info@barberusa.com; www.barberusa.com

Allianza Hair Salon: Yiannis Karimalis, hairstylist; 29199 Northwestern Highway, Southfield, MI 48034; (248) 356-3230

Allure Day Spa and Hair Design: Valerie Estrada, master stylist; 139 East
55th Street, New York, NY 10022; (212) 644-5500;
www.alluredayspa.com

Arrojo Cutler Salon: Marcello, hair colorist; 115 East 57th Street,
New York, NY 10022; (212) 308-3838

Aveda: Pat Peterson, director of research and development; (800) 328-0849,
www.aveda.com

Avon Salon & Spa: Trump Tower, 725 Fifth Avenue at 56th St., New York, NY,
10022; (212) 755-AVON: Brad Johns, artistic director, celebrity colorist;
Gayle Reichler, nutritionist; Joelle, senior stylist; Ted Giza, senior stylist;
www.avonsalonandspa.com

Barry Hendrickson's Bitz-n-Pieces: 1841 Broadway, New York, NY, 10023;
(212) 397-0711: Edward James Maloney, assistant manager and stylist

Chattem Chemicals: Mike Davies, research and development manager for
Chattem, the makers of Ultraswim shampoo and conditioner;
www.chattemchemicals.com

Conair: Paulette Heller, director of marketing for hair dryers;
(203) 351-9000; www.conair.com

David Kinigson: New York–based hairstylist, creative consultant,
and educator; (561) 416-7479

Ethnicsoul.com: Offering black hair care; 601 West 26th Street,
14th Floor, Suite 8, New York, NY 10001

Eufora International: Haim Knister, artist; contact Haim Limited Salon at
(858) 259-0559; www.eufora.net

Filles et Garçons Salons: 673 Lexington Avenue, New York, NY 10022; (212) 688-6655

Galderma: Mary Madden, senior product manager; (871) 961-5000; www.galderma.com

Lynn Glaze: A John Paul Mitchell Systems and Rogaine trainer, and owner of Sheer Reflections: The Salon, 282 Edgewood Drive, Pineville, LA 71360; (318) 442-TATA or e-mail: sheerreflections@aol.com

Hans Schwarzkopf Professional: Bob Siebert, national director of education; (310) 641-4600 ext. 180; www.schwarzkopf.com

Hill Dermaceuticals: The makers of Derma-Smoothe FS: Maria Darnell, director of information services; (800) 344-5707; www.hillderm.com

Jean-Pierre Creations: Elizabeth Manoughian, president; (877) JPIERRE; www.jean-pierre-creations.com

John Sahag Salon: John Sahag, owner; 425 Madison Avenue, New York, NY 10017; (212) 750-7772

Joseph Martin Salon: Doug MacIntosh, colorist; 717 Madison Avenue, New York, NY 10021; (212) 838-3150; www.josephmartin.com

Laura Geller Make-up Studio: Laura Geller, owner; 1044 Lexington Avenue, New York, NY 10021; (212) 570-5477; www.laurageller.com

L'Oréal: Julia Youssef, technical center director; 575 FifthAvenue, New York, NY 10017; (212) 818-1500 ext. 4422; www.loreal.com

Mark Garrison Salon: Mark Garrison, owner; 820 Madison Avenue, New York, NY 10021; (212) 570-2455; www.markgarrisonsalon.com

Mason Pearson: Robert Sansone, national sales director; 7 Main Street, East Rockaway, NY 11518; (516) 599-1776; www.masonpearson.com

McNeil Consumer & Specialty Pharmaceuticals: A Johnson & Johnson Company. They are the makers of Nizoral A-D; 7050 Camp Hill Road, Fort Washington, PA 19034; (800) 962-5357; www.jnj.com

Minardi Salon: Carmine and Beth Minardi, owners; 29 East 61st Street, New York, NY, 10021; (212) 308-1711 or e-mail: minardinyc@aol.com

Oribe Salons: Oribe, owner and consulting stylist to Oribe Salons and L'Oréal; 691 5th Avenue, 10th Floor, New York, NY 10022; (212) 319-3910; www.oribesalon.com

Oscar Bond Salon: Oscar Bond, owner; 42 Wooster Street, New York, NY 10013; (212) 334-3777; www.oscarbondsalon.com

Osis Hair Care Products: Andrea Wentz, brand manager; 6047 Bristol Parkway, Suite 200, Culver City, CA 90230; (800) 707-9997; available at www.schwarzkopf.com and at www.salon-collective.co.uk

Ouidad: Ouidad, curly hair specialist; 846 Seventh Avenue, 5th Floor, New York, NY 10019; (212) 333-7577; www.ouidad.com

Pantene: Cheri McMaster, senior scientist in product development and consumer habits; Procter & Gamble Co., 1511 Reed Hartman Highway, Cincinnati, OH 45241; (513) 626-2500; www.pantene.com

Paul Labrecque Salon and Spa: Paul Labrecque, owner; 160 Columbus Avenue at The Reebok Sports Club NY, New York, NY 10023; (212) 595-0099; www.paullabrecque.com

Progressive Beauty Brands: Rick Goldberg, head coach; www.progressivebeautybrands.com

Susan Rabin: M.A., New York–based psychologist. Rabin has a masters degree in counseling, is the author of *101 Ways to Flirt*, and is the director of School of Flirting; (212) 369-3311; www.schoolofflirting.com

TLC Inc.: Christina Pearson, executive director for the national nonprofit education and resource center devoted to advancing understanding of trichotillomania (TTM), or compulsive hair-pulling; 303 Potrero Street, Suite 51,Santa Cruz, CA 95060; (831) 457-1004 or (831) 426-4383 (fax); www.trich.org

TwoDo Salon: Megan Gordon, owner and head colorist; 210 W. 82nd Street, New York, NY 10024; (212) 787-1277; www.twodo.com

Unilever Home and Personal Care, Rolling Meadows, IL: Joanne Crudele, senior development manager for Salon Selectives, Finesse, Thermasilk, and Suave, among other brands; (847) 734-3712; www.unilever.com

Yves Durif Salon: Yves Durif, owner; 130 East 65th Street, New York, NY 10021; (212) 452-0954; www.citysearch.com

Dedicated Doctors

There are qualified medical experts that can help you with all your hair-thinning and loss problems in most cities and towns. Here are some respected physicians from around the country:

California

Rosanelli, Tom, M.D., chairman of the American Society of Hair Restoration Surgery, a fellow of the American Academy of Cosmetic Surgery, and one of the founders and faculty members of the International Society of Hair Restoration Surgery,
(415) 931-9881,
website: www.rosanelli.com

Florida

Bissoon, Lionel, D.O., a mesotherapist based in Hollywood, California, New York City, and West Palm Beach, FL,
(561) 655-3031

Epstein, Jeffrey, M.D., F.A.C.S., a doctor in private practice in Miami, FL,
(305) 666-1774

New Jersey

Peritz, Mitch J., D.C., C.C.N., in private practice in New York and New Jersey,
(212) 995-5525

Glasgold, Mark, M.D., a facial and plastic surgeon, based
in Highland Park, NJ,
(732) 846-6540

New York

Baldwin, Hilary, M.D., associate professor of dermatology at the State
University of New York at Downstate Medical Center,
(718) 270-1229

Denese, Adrienne, M.D., Ph.D., a specialist in antiaging medicine in private
practice in New York City, NY,
(212) 517-6600

Guida, Robert, M.D., director of facial and plastic surgery at New York
Hospital Cornell Medical Center, New York City, NY,
(212) 871-0900

Lebwohl, Mark, M.D., professor and chairman of the department
of dermatology at Mount Sinai School of Medicine, New York City, NY,
(212) 876-7199

Lewis, Amy Beth, M.D., assistant clinical professor of dermatology at
Downstate Medical Center and a New York City, NY—based dermatologist,
(212) 288-6133

Peck, Valerie, M.D., clinical associate professor of medicine, department of
endocrinology, New York University Medical Center, New York City, NY,
(212) 263-7434

Romo, Thomas III, M.D., director of facial, plastic, and reconstructive surgery at Lenox Hill Hospital in New York City and Manhattan Eye, Ear and Throat in New York City, NY,
(212) 288-1500

Victor, Steven, M.D., New York City, NY–based hair transplant surgeon,
(212) 249-3050

Ohio

Bergfeld, Wilma F., M.D., F.A.C.P., head of clinical research, department of dermatology and pathology, The Cleveland Clinic, in Cleveland, OH,
(216) 444-5722

Texas

Arem, Ridha, M.D., in private practice in Houston, TX,
(713) 790-0102

Organizations

Need more info? There are plenty of places to contact. Here, a handful of organizations dedicated to answering your hair-loss questions and other related issues.

American Academy of Cosmetic Surgery
737 N. Michigan Avenue, Suite 820
Chicago, IL 60611
(312) 981-6760
www.cosmeticsurgery.org

American Academy of Dermatology (AAD)
930 Woodfield Road
PO Box 4014
Schaumburg, IL 60173-4014
Phone: (847) 330-0230
www.aad.org

American Academy of Facial, Plastic and Reconstructive Surgery
310 S. Henry Street
Alexandria, VA 22314
(703) 299-9291
www.facial-plastic-surgery.org

American Association of Pharmaceutical Scientists (AAPS)
2107 Wilson Boulevard, Suite 700
Arlington, VA 22201-3046
Phone: (703) 243-2800
www.aaps.org

American Board of Facial, Plastic and Reconstructive Surgery
115C South Saint Asaph Street
Alexandria, VA 22314
(703) 549-3223
www.abfprs.org

American Cancer Society
1599 Clifton Road, NE
Atlanta, GA 30329
(404) 320-3333
(800) 227-2345
www.cancer.org

American College of Surgeons (ACS)
633 North Saint Clair Street
Chicago, IL 60611-3211
(312) 202-5000
www.facs.org

American Hair Loss Council
125 Seventh Street, Suite 625
Pittsburgh, PA 15222
(412) 765-3666
(412) 765-3669 (fax)
www.ahlc.org

American Medical Association (AMA)
515 North State Street
Chicago, IL 60610
Phone: (312) 464-5000
www.ama-assn.org

American Medical Women's Association (AMWA)
801 N. FairFax Street, Suite 400
Alexandria, VA 22314
Phone: (703) 838-0500
www.amwa-doc.org

American Pharmaceutical Association (APhA)
2215 Constitution Avenue, NW
Washington, DC 20037-2985
Phone: (202) 628-4410
www.aphanet.org

American Psychiatric Association (APA)
1400 K Street, NW
Washington, DC 20005
Phone: (888) 357-7924
www.psych.org

American Skin Association
346 Park Avenue South, 4th Floor
New York, NY 10010
(212) 889-4858 or (800) 499-SKIN
www.skinassn.org

American Society for Aesthetic Plastic Surgery
36 West 44th Street, Suite 630
New York, NY 10036
(212) 921-0500
(888) 272-7711
www.surgery.org

American Society for Dermatologic Surgery
5550 Meadowbrook Drive, Suite 120
Rolling Meadows, IL 60008
(847) 956-0900
www.asds-net.org

American Society of Hair Restoration Surgery (a division of the American
Academy of Cosmetic Surgery)
737 North Michigan Avenue, Suite 820
Chicago, IL 60611-6659
(312) 981-6771
www.cosmeticsurgery.org

American Society of Plastic Surgeons
444 East Algonquin Road
Arlington Heights, IL 60005
(847) 228-9900
(888) 752-7842
www.plasticsurgery.com

Cancer Research Institute
681 Fifth Avenue
New York, NY 10022
Phone: (212) 688-7515 or (800) 99-CANCER
www.cancerresearch.org

Federation of State Medical Boards
Federation Place
400 Fuller Wiser Road, Suite 300
Euless, TX 76039-3855
Phone: (817) 868-4000
www.fsmb.org

National Alopecia Areata Foundation (NAAF)
14 Mitchell Boulevard
PO Box 150760
San Rafael, CA 94903
(415) 456-4644 or
(415) 472-3780
www.alopeciaareata.com

National Eczema Association for Science and Education
6600 SW 92nd Avenue, Suite 230
Portland, OR 97223-0704
(503) 228-4430 or (800) 818-7546
www.nationaleczema.org

National Psoriasis Foundation
6600 SW 92nd Avenue, Suite 300
Portland, OR 97223-7195
(503) 244-7404
(800) 723-9166
E-mail: getinfo@npfusa.org
www.psoriasis.org

National Women's Health Information Center (NWHIC)
8550 Arlington Boulevard, Suite 300
Fairfax, VA 22030
(800) 994-WOMAN
(888) 220-5446
www.4woman.gov

Pharmaceutical Research and Manufacturers of America
1100 Fifteenth Street, NW, Suite 900
Washington, DC 20005
(202) 835-3400
www.phrma.org

Society for Women's Health Research
1828 L Street, NW, Suite 625
Washington, DC 20036
(202) 223-8224;
Fax: (202) 833-3472
www.womens-health.org

The Women's Institute for Fine and Thinning Hair (sponsored by Rogaine)
(800) 764-2463 or
(877) 554-HAIR (for Women's Institute consumer brochures)
www.womenshairinstitute.com

Journals

These medical journals can provide up-to-the-minute news on hair problems, thinning, and loss.

British Medical Journal
BMJ Publishing Group (a division of the British Medical Association—BMA)
www.bmj.com

Depression and Bipolar Support Alliance Brochures and Publications
Depression and Bipolar Support Alliance (formerly the National Depressive and Manic Depressive Association—DMDA)
www.ndmda.org

Hair Loss Journal
American Hair Loss Council
www.ahlc.org

Journal of the American Medical Association (JAMA)
American Medical Association
www.jama.ama-assn.org

National Psoriasis Foundation Bulletin
National Psoriasis Foundation
www.psoriasis.org

Books

There's a library full of books on hair care. Each will supplement the information you find in *The Hair Bible*, a unique hair guide for women.

Andre Talks Hair
by Andre Walker with Teresa Wiltz
Simon & Schuster, New York; 1997

Beauty, The New Basics
by Rona Berg
Workman Publishing Company, New York; 2001

Beauty: The Twentieth Century
by Jacqueline Demornex and Fabienne Russo
Universe Publishing, New York; 2000

D.I.Y. (Do-It-Yourself) Beauty
by Karen W. Bressler and Susan Redstone
Penguin Putnam Books, New York; 2000

Hair: An Owner's Handbook
by Philip Kingsley
Aurum Press Limited, London; 1995

Home Spa: Recipes and Techniques to Restore and Refresh
by Manine Rosa Golden
Abbeville Press Inc., New York; 1997

Mother Nature's Guide to Vibrant Beauty and Health
by Myra Cameron and Theresa Foy DiGeronimo
Prentice Hall, Paramus, NJ; 1997

SalonOvations Public Relations for the Salon
by Jayne Morehouse
Milady Publishing Co., Albany, NY; 1996

Skin Deep: An A–Z of Skin Disorders, Treatments and Health
by Carol A. Turkington and Jeffrey S. Dover, M.D.
Facts on File, Inc., New York; 1998

Skin Sense: A Dermatologist's Complete Guide to Your Family's Skin Care
by Garry Gewirtzman, M.D.,
Frederick Fell Publishers, Hollywood, FL; 1993

*The Bald Truth: The First Complete Guide to Preventing
and Treating Hair Loss*
by Spencer David Kobren
Pocket Books, New York; 1998

*The Wrinkle Cure: Unlock the Power of Cosmeceuticals for Supple,
Youthful Skin*
by Nicholas Perricone, M.D.
Warner Books, New York; 2001

Trade Publications

Want to keep up to date on the latest hair looks? Check out these maga-zine and journals dedicated to bringing you trends, tips, and styling tech-niques.

American Salon
1 Park Avenue
New York, NY 10016
(212) 951-6600
www.americansalongroup.com

Harris Publications, Inc.
1115 Broadway
New York, NY 10010
(212) 807-7100

Modern Salon
370 Lexington Avenue
Suite 1206
New York, NY 10017
(212) 682-7777
www.modernsalon.com

Salon News
Fairchild Publications
7 West 34th Street
New York, NY 10001
(212) 630-3547

Sophisticate's Hairstyle Guides
875 North Michigan Avenue
Suite 3434
Chicago, IL 60611
(312) 266-8680

Hair Salons

Looking for a great place to go to get your hair into shape? Find a salon in your city that can give your hair a look you'll love.

Atlanta

Don and Sylvia Shaw Salon and Spa
4400 Ashford Dunwoody Road
Suite 4010
Atlanta, GA 30346
(770) 393-8303
www.donshaw.com

Scott Cole David King Salon
2859 Piedmont Road NE
Atlanta, GA 30305
(404) 237-4970

Studio Oliver
789 Argonne Avenue
Atlanta, GA
(404) 607-9757

Boston

Diego
143 Newbury Street
Boston, MA 02116
(617) 262-5003

Niall Roberts Hair Studio
253 Newbury Street
Boston, MA 02116
(617) 536-7243

Salon Mario Russo
9 Newbury Street
Boston, MA 02116
(617) 424-6676
www.mariorusso.com

Chicago

Mario Tricoci Hair Salon & Day Spa
900 North Michigan Avenue
Chicago, IL 60611
(312) 915-0960
www.tricoci.com

Maxine Ltd.
712 North Rush Street
Chicago, IL 60611
(312) 751-1511
www.maxinesalon.com

Tiffani Kim Institute
310 W. Superior Street
Chicago, IL 60610
(312) 943-8777
www.tiffanikiminstitute.com

Connecticut

Adam Broderick Salon & Spa
89 Danbury Road
Ridgefield, CT 06877
(203) 431-3994 or (800) 438-3834
www.adambroderick.com

De Berardinis Salon and Day Spa
124 Greenwich Avenue
Greenwich, CT 06830
(203) 622-4247
www.deberardinis.com

Noelle Day Spa
1100 High Ridge Road
Stamford, CT 06905
(203) 322-3445

Houston

Jon Henderson Salon
4621 Montrose, Suite B240
Houston, TX 77006
(713) 522-1585

Solution
1920 Brun Street
Houston, TX 77019
(713) 526-4545
e-mail: solution@net1.net

Las Vegas

The Robert Cromeans Salon
Mandalay Bay
3950 Las Vegas Boulevard South
Las Vegas, NV 89119
(702) 632-6130

Los Angeles

Beauty Bar
1638 N. Cahuenga Boulevard
Hollywood, CA 90028
(323) 464-7676
www.beautybar.com

ChopChop Salon Gallery
830 N. La Brea
Hollywood, CA 90048
(323) 464-8100

Equinox
1433 6th Street
Santa Monica, CA 90401
(310) 394-7563

Frédéric Fekkai
Beverly Hills Salon & Boutique
440 N. Rodeo Drive
Beverly Hills, CA 90210
(310) 777-8700

Goodform Hollywood
727 North Fairfax Avenue
Los Angeles, CA 90046
(323) 658-8585

Hair America (at the Art Luna Salon)
8930 Keith Avenue
West Hollywood, CA 90069
(310) 247-9092

JosephMartin Salon
421 North Rodeo Drive
Beverly Hills, CA 90210
(310) 274-0109
www.josephmartin.com

Prive Salon
7373 Beverly Boulevard
Los Angeles, CA 90036
(323) 931-5559

Sally Hershberger at John Frieda
8440 Melrose Place
Los Angeles, CA 90069
(323) 653-4040

Steam
314 N. Harper Avenue
Los Angeles, CA 90048
(323) 966-0024

Vidal Sassoon
9403 Little Santa Monica Boulevard
Beverly Hills, CA 90210
(310) 274-8791

Louisiana

Sheer Reflections: The Salon
282 Edgewood Drive
Pineville, LA 71360
(800) 843-7256
e-mail: sheerreflections@aol.com

Michigan

Allianza Salon
29199 Northwestern Highway
Southfield, MI 48034
(248) 356-3230

Jeffrey Michael Powers Beauty Spa
206 S. Fifth Avenue, Suite 300
Ann Arbor, MI 48104
(734) 996-5585

Miami

Stella Salon
404 Washington Avenue, Suite 150
Miami Beach, FL 33139
(305) 532-0024

New York

Allure Day Spa and Hair Design
139 East 55th Street
New York, NY 10022
(212) 644-5500

Avon Salon & Spa
Trump Tower
725 Fifth Avenue
New York, NY 10022
(212) 755-AVON
(888) 577-AVON
www.avonsalonandspa.com

Bumble and Bumble
146 East 56th Street
New York, NY 10022
(212) 521-6500
(800) 7BUMBLE
www.bumbleandbumble.com

Coppola Salon
746 Madison Avenue
New York, NY 10021
(212) 988-9404

Devachan
560 Broadway
New York, NY 10012
(212) 274-8686

Filles et Garçons Salons
673 Lexington Avenue at 56th Street; (212) 688-6655
50 West 55 Street; (212) 586-6585
760 Third Avenue at 47th Street; (212) 486-6943
New York, NY 10019

Frédéric Fekkai Beauté de Provence
15 East 57th Street
New York, NY 10022
(212) 753-9500

Garren New York (at Henri Bendel)
712 Fifth Avenue, 3rd Floor
New York, NY 10019
(212) 841-9400
www.garrennewyork.com

Gil Ferrer Salon
21 East 74th Street
New York, NY 10021
(212) 535-3543

John Frieda Salon
797 Madison Avenue, 2nd Floor
New York, NY 10021
(212) 879-1000

John Sahag Workshop
425 Madison Avenue, 2nd Floor
New York, NY 10017
(212) 750-7772

Lépine New York
667 Madison Avenue, (at 61st Street)
New York, NY 10021
(212) 355-4247
www.lepinehair.com

Louis Licari
693 Fifth Avenue
New York, NY 10023
(212) 758-2090

Mark Garrison Salon
820 Madison Avenue
New York, NY 10021
(212) 570-2455

Maximus
2075 Merrick Road
Merrick, NY 11566
(516) 623-4180

Minardi Salon
29 East 61st Street
New York, NY 10021
(212) 308-1711

Nubest & Co. Hair Salon
1482 Northern Boulevard
Manhasset, NY 11030
(516) 627-9444

Oscar Blandi Salon
768 Fifth Avenue, (at The Plaza Hotel)
New York, NY 10019
(212) 573-7930

Oscar Bond Salon
42 Wooster Street
New York, NY 10013
(212) 334-3777
www.oscarbondsalon.com

Ouidad Salon
846 Seventh Avenue, 5th Floor
New York, NY 10019
(212) 333-7577
(800) 677-HAIR
www.ouidad.com

Paul Labrecque Salon
160 Columbus Avenue
New York, NY 10023
(212) 595-0099
www.paullabrecque.com

Scott J. Aveda Lifestyle Salon and Spa
2415 Main Street
Bridgehampton, NY 11932
(631) 537-6696

Stephen Knoll
625 Madison Avenue, 2nd Floor
New York, NY 10022
(212) 421-0100

TwoDo Salon
210 West 82nd Street
New York, NY 10024
(212) 787-1277

Uliana Hair & Makeup Studio
321 East 9th Street
New York, NY 10011
(212) 475-4302

Vidal Sassoon
Uptown Address:
730 Fifth Avenue, 2nd Floor
New York, NY 10019
(212) 535-9200
Downtown Address:
90 Fifth Avenue
New York NY 10011
(212) 229-2200

Warren-Tricomi
16 West 57th Street, 4th Floor
New York, NY 10019
(212) 262-8899

Yves Durif Salon
130 East 65th Street
New York, NY 10021
(212) 452-0954

Philadelphia

Adolf Biecker Salon, Spa and Healthclub
210 West Rittenhouse Square, 3rd Floor
Philadelphia, PA 19103
(215) 735-6404

Richard Nicholas Hair Studio, Inc.
1716 Sansom Street
Philadelphia, PA 19103
(215) 567-4790

Phoenix

Carsten Phoenix
4415 E. Indian School Road
Phoenix, AZ 85018
(602) 840-4240
www.carsteninstituteandsalons.com

San Francisco

Yosh for Hair/Gina Khan
173 Maiden Lane
San Francisco, CA 94108
(415) 989-7704

Seattle

Marco Two Union Square
601 Union Street, Suite 220
Seattle, WA 98101
(206) 628-8881

Phase 3
99 Blanchard Street
Seattle, WA 98121
(206) 728-9933

Virginia

Bubbles Salon and Spa
1143 Emmet Street N
Charlottesville, VA 22901
(434) 293-2667
www.bubblessalon.com

Vidal Sassoon
Tyson Galleria
1855 G International Drive
McLean, VA 22102
(703) 448-9884
www.vidalsassoon.com

Washington, D.C.

Molecule
1800 M Street, NW
Washington, D.C. 20036
(202) 822-1588
www.moleculesalon.com

Personal Resources

Index

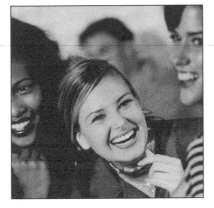

Notes

9/10 (27) 6/10
9/15 (30) 1/15

Notes